GUIDE for CANCER SUPPORTERS

This book is available to you without charge with the belief that it will truly help you, the supporter, to improve the quality of life of the cancer patient and increase their chances of successfully fighting their disease. After you have read the book, please give it to another supporter. If you are unable to do this, please give it to a library or minister so that they may loan it to someone it can help.

We would appreciate hearing your feelings after you read this book. Drop us a note. We care about you and the one near to you with cancer.

Annette Bloch
R.A Bloch Cancer Foundation
One H&R Block Way
Kansas City, MO 64105
Phone: 800-433-0464 or
        816-854-5050

Annette and Richard Bloch

Guide for Cancer Supporters

STEP-BY-STEP WAYS TO HELP A RELATIVE OR FRIEND FIGHT CANCER

Note:

In this book, the patient is referred to as "they" or "themself." This was done to alleviate the awkward "he or she" or "himself or herself." Also, the authors arbitrarily refer to the physician as "he" and the supporter as "you" or "she."

We have periodically revised the book to make sure that the statistics and treatments are current. In this edition, the University of Kansas Cancer Center staff aided us in updating the contents. We want to especially thank Lynn Marzinski, RN MSN AOCN CNS for her work on this revision.

Dedication

This book is dedicated to our three daughters who were by our side continuously during the year of strenuous treatments, to our wonderful friends who were with us when we needed them, to the wonderful nurses, social workers, ministers and rabbis and other care givers who were an integral part of our support group, and particularly to "our" doctor who cured Dick from lung cancer. He knew the odds but he also knew the wisdom of bringing in specialists in the various disciplines to do what they are best at. He was like the conductor of a great orchestra. Not only did he cure Dick but he taught him a great deal about cancer, life and living along the way. He allowed Dick to fight to live rather than to wait to die. There is no doubt that he, like every other oncologist, fails to successfully treat a patient from time to time. I hope he realizes that he gave them true hope in trying to fight and restored a quality to their life, the most important factor there is.

A physician who will try to help a patient makes the support system possible.

Table of Contents

Table of Contents

Foreword

by Jimmie C. Holland, M.D., Director Emeritus, Psychiatric Oncology, Memorial Sloan-Kettering Cancer Center

When cancer is diagnosed, it is not only the person diagnosed who experiences concerns about the future – but also the relatives and friends. In fact, studies have shown that levels of distress are just as high in the next of kin as in the patient! That is why we think of cancer as a "family" disease and recognize that support is needed by the family members as well as the patient. Other studies show that helping the spouse of a cancer patient cope better has a substantial effect upon the patient's ability to cope and can work like a "ripple" effect.

The best way to counter that initial over-whelming fear which accompanies a diagnosis of cancer is to get the best information available about cancer and its treatment and to begin to cope with the psychological impact. The need for commitment to a course of positive action is an important way of beginning to cope.

"What can I read?" is an increasingly common question. Advice for the caring family and friends has been sparse but this valuable little book begins to fill the gap. It carries the added weight of having been written by the Blochs who speak with the voice of experience - and who share "how it felt" to be given a three-month prognosis. The commitment to finding treatment and not giving up is a success story we all benefit from today.

Part I is a powerful review of the "what it feels like" of cancer. Written for the healthy spouses of patients, it gives important practical advice about helping the ill spouse. An important message is the value of providing support and access to good information, but not at the expense of taking the decision making away and respecting the person's individuality and need for independence. We live in an era when some books suggest there is only **one** correct way (their way) to face cancer and those who don't are doomed. The Blochs encourage respect for each person's coping style and their right to use it. The spouse is an important force in making the patient feel guilty for not using a particular method, or in feeling empowered and confident because they feel supported by their spouse in their handling of their cancer.

More attention to "helping the helper" is needed and hence, the value of this book, especially for spouses. The spouse must simultaneously support the patient, manage the home and family, make the living, manage the insurance forms, arrange visits to the doctor, share discussions about cancer, and answer all the well-meaning calls asking "How is Joe?" but rarely, "How are **you**?" The strains, borne without much recognition or praise, are difficult. More of our efforts must be directed to assure the spouse copes, since so much rests on the healthy adult. The Well Spouse Foundation is a self help organization which has developed out of awareness of this need.

Part II is an excellent brief introduction to cancer therapies which is useful as one hears these words for the first time in a personal context.

Part III is directed to the casual friend who suffers from "Do I visit my friend with cancer?" "What do I say?" "Will it be the wrong thing?" Advice to reduce self-consciousness and affirmation of the need to keep ties which antedate the onset of cancer come through clearly in this practical guide.

Last, biographies sometimes tell more than all the "do as I say" advice reveals. Dick Bloch's biography is a powerful "call to arms" at the book's end, sharing how one couple coped and won. It is well worth emulating!

Introduction

Often when a person hears of someone near and dear to them being told they have cancer, their first reactions are – what can I do, how do I treat them, what do I say to them? Possibly the worst thing you can do is to do nothing, ignore the situation and avoid any discussion for fear of saying and doing the wrong thing.

This book is written to help you understand the facts about cancer, its probable effects on the patient and their likely reactions to the diagnosis. This will enable you to better fill the needs of the patient, whether your relationship is casual or you are the primary supporter or somewhere in between.

Part I is for the primary caregiver detailing the actions to take to truly help the cancer patient. Part II is a brief description of medical treatments available to a cancer patient and definitions, so you can educate yourself and be able to discuss them intelligently. Part III is designed to allow the casual supporter to be comfortable and constructive.

Chapter 9 includes a check list of specific helpful hints for the primary supporter in taking care of oneself.

If you are the primary supporter, such as a spouse, parent, child or closest friend, you will want to thoroughly read Part I and possibly Part II. If you are a casual acquaintance, you will want to concentrate on Part III.

The American Cancer Society predicts that one out of every three Americans will be stricken with cancer. Nearly every family will be affected. The chances are sooner or later you will appreciate suggestions on how to approach and communicate with the patient and be truly helpful as well as how to cope yourself.

The fundamental thread to remember is that the patient is a living being. The diagnosis of disease may have changed their focus, but it has not changed their likes and dislikes. Like every human being, they have interests they want to continue sharing. Be there for them and with them.

Sorrow is for the dead. Concern and caring is for the living. The worst thing you can do is to avoid the patient. Be with them. Your actions do not have to be negative, submissive or passive. They should be positive, active and helpful.

Remember, cancer is a word, not a sentence.

Understanding the Patient 1

This book is about actions! Actions you can take from the very beginning and continue all the way through a cancer patient's recovery. What is important is to do the things that will really help the patient. Make them feel better now and in the long run. Try to help them have a better chance of succeeding in the fight against their disease.

In order to be a true helper, start out trying to understand how the patient feels. That is not what they say or how they act, but their true deep down feelings. To do this you must understand what they are going through.

They have been told they have cancer. It is impossible to appreciate the gravity of that short statement if you have not yourself been told this. Cancer is the most feared disease in America. All our life, we have been raised to understand that cancer kills. We have been told it is a horrible disease accompanied by pain, suffering and treatments that are probably worse than the disease itself. Even though we might not recall them at the moment, our subconscious recalls individuals who have had cancer, all of whom suffered and died. Supposedly cancer means pain and imminent death.

This is probably the first time the patient has had to seriously face their own mortality. Sure, we're all told from childhood that someday we will all die. But that is someday. Now they are told that someday is here. Wow! No matter what the age of the patient, it is like trying to get a child to leave a game arcade. They want to play just one more game. It is not unnatural to think about dying, but the important thing is to concentrate on living.

How suddenly their whole life changed! Cancer is often discovered by a doctor looking for the cause of a minor complaint or accidentally on a routine physical exam. One instant they are perfect or have a small complaint and the next they are told they have cancer, a term they know to be painfully fatal.

Next come all the psychological reactions. These are not isolated or occasional events, but in talking with cancer patients, happen universally to all those diagnosed. "Why me?" "What did I do to cause this?" "What did I do to deserve this?" "Whom did I hurt?" "Where did I go wrong?" "So many others will be hurt because I have failed." The guilt trip is immense!

"I'm so angry." "Why now?" "Just when

things are starting to break for me." "Just when I'm starting to succeed." "Just when I'm starting to have fun." "There's no justice in this world." This anger is often vented at the health care system, at oneself and those who help the patient including the supporter.

Talk about being scared! From every standpoint this is the most frightening thing that has ever happened. What is being scared? It is not knowing the future and fearing what it might be. And that fear has no bounds. It runs from death to treatments, to incapacity, to not knowing where to turn, to financial burden, to exposing their body and their thoughts, to who is going to care for others, to everything imaginable.

And isolation! "No one else has such a bad problem." "Everyone else is so happy and going about their business." "This is so rare." "I don't want to burden others with my problems." "I don't believe anyone else wants to be around me." "No one really cares." "I can't count on anyone." "They give me lip service but they really don't mean it." "I can't trust anyone anymore." "Maybe I can curl up in a corner and it will go away."

Then there is denial. "They made a mistake." "I really don't have cancer." "You read about these medical errors all the time." "I feel too good to be that sick." "Maybe the doctor got the wrong

X-rays or maybe he misread them." "Should I just forget about it and see what happens?"

The list goes on and on. These are the universal feelings of every individual we have talked with who had cancer. These feelings are normal, natural and expected. A supporter will have comparable reactions. It's okay, and we should not feel guilty about it.

Whether the outlook for recovery is good or poor, the days go by, one at a time, and the patient and family must learn to live each one. It's not always easy. On learning the diagnosis, some decide that death is inevitable, and there is nothing to do but give up and wait. They are not the first to feel that way.

Orville Kelly, a newspaperman, described his initial battle with the specter of death. "I began to isolate myself from the rest of the world. I spent much time in bed, even though I was physically able to walk and drive. I thought about my own impending funeral and it made me very sad." These feelings continued from his first hospitalization through the first outpatient chemotherapy treatment. On the way home from that treatment, he was haunted by memories of the happy past, when "everything was all right."

Then it occurred to Kelly, "I wasn't dead yet.

I was able to drive my automobile. Why couldn't I return home to barbecue ribs?" He did, that very night. He began to talk to his wife and children about his fears and anxieties. And he became so frustrated at the feelings he had kept locked up inside himself that he wrote the newspaper article that led to the founding of Make Today Count, a mutual help group.

Each person must work through individual feelings of possible death, fear and isolation in his or her own good time. It is hard to overcome these feelings if they are never confronted head on, but it is an ongoing struggle. One day brings feelings of confidence, the next day despair. Many people find it helps considerably if they strive to return, both as individuals and as a family, to their normal lives.

Only when you thoroughly understand the patient, can you help. They are out there cold and alone in a totally strange place they have never seen and don't know where they are going or what they are supposed to do. With that in mind, where do you start out to help?

First, understand some truisms about cancer:

1. Cancer is the most curable of all chronic diseases.

2. There is no type of cancer for which there are no treatments!

3. There is no type of cancer from which some people have not been cured!

Next, make a list of things not to do:

1. Sympathy for the sake of sympathy doesn't help anyone. Show your compassion followed by a positive, constructive statement. An example would be, "I'm sorry you have to go through this ordeal, but be grateful that it was caught at this time and medical treatments have advanced so greatly."

2. Tears and sorrow are for the dead, not the living. When you are with the patient, cry with the patient, not for the patient. It can lead to meaningful conversations.

3. Never lie or state anything that is not a fact. It will ruin your credibility and come back to haunt you. For example, never say "I know you are going to get well." You can't possibly know that and the patient realizes it. Therefore, anything else you said with that would be ignored. However, it is possible to

state any negative comments in a positive and constructive vein. "It's very serious, but we're going to do everything in our power to beat it" is an example.

4. There are no secrets from a cancer patient. Be totally open and honest, but with tact and optimism.

5. Do not classify in your own mind the patient as a statistic. This can cause you to harbor false feelings and your feelings have a way of coming through.

6. Do not encourage a feeling of futility. The patient's actions might make a difference in the outcome and will make a difference in the quality of their life.

7. Do not discourage work, prayer, exercise or diet.

8. Do not make a prognosis.

9. Do not make decisions for the patient that the patient is capable of making.

10. Do not fail to express love, caring and concern. Let the patient know how much you are hurting and the anger you are also feeling.

To summarize, your friend or relative is going through a traumatic time in their life. They don't need your sympathy. They need your help, support and direction. Do not say, "John, it is so terrible" or "John, it's such a shame." Do say, "John, we're going to do everything we can to try to get you healthy again."

Making a Decision to Fight 2

The greatest single thing that you can do to help a cancer patient is to convince them to make up their mind to really fight it. They must, on their own, make the commitment that they will do everything in their power to fight their disease. No exceptions. Nothing halfway. Nothing for the sake of ease or convenience. Everything! Nothing short of it. When they have done this, they have accomplished the most difficult thing they will have to accomplish throughout their entire treatment. And it doesn't matter how serious or how minor they are led to believe their cancer is.

If it is minor, great. Their commitment should not be difficult to abide by. If they are told they are going to die in 3 months or 3 years or whatever, their commitment is that much more vital. There are a lot of "terminal" people alive, healthy and cancer free. There is no type of cancer for which there is no treatment. There is no type of cancer from which some people have not been cured.

The statistics for the worst kind of cancer show a 2% survival, meaning 20 out of 1,000 beat it. We have received numerous letters from individuals stating they were told they were terminal and are now cancer free.

To give up requires no commitment. They can stay in the comfort of their own lifestyle. Fighting means a complete change of lifestyle, absolutely leaving their comfort zone. There will be doctors doing things they might not like. There will be lots of work for them to do. There might even be some pain and suffering and, certainly, lots of new and unexpected experiences. They must decide that the end is worth the means because they are the only one who can do it. No one else can do it for them. There is no half way. It's all the way. But when it is all said and done, no matter what the results, I've never met anyone who felt it was not the best way. See that they go for it with no second thoughts or regrets. Remember, once they have made the commitment, everything else is relatively easy. There will be pleasant experiences. There will be unpleasant experiences. But I can promise you nothing they will do will be as difficult as making the decision to make the commitment.

You will probably find your friend or relative saying, "I'm going to make it," or "Sure, I'll do everything needed." But that is a long way from making the commitment. Without a commitment, every step of the way is another torturous decision. Should I do this? Should I do that? Is this worth the time or effort? With the commitment, there is only one question: will it help me? If it might, then they do it. If it won't help, they don't do it. You can help the patient by seeing that they make this commitment and then help them stick to it. At the initial diagnosis, my wife cried in the visitor's waiting room. When I came to in the recovery room with my wife there and was told I had cancer, I cried. My wife said in determination, "Dick, we're going to beat this. Give me your word and promise that you and I are going to fight and beat this thing together." I did and I stopped crying right there.

A year of tough treatments later, when an X-ray unexpectedly showed what appeared like a recurrence, I said to my wife that I could not go through this all over again. She again said in a tough and determined voice, "You can, and you will if you have to." I agreed and was willing to start all over again if need be. Thank goodness this time the commitment was not necessary because it was scar tissue and not a recurrence, but I would have had I needed to.

I was diagnosed on a Wednesday. Being told I was terminal by one doctor, I first talked to a new doctor 900 miles away at 11 pm. He suggested I come on Thursday, and they would examine me on Friday. They were closed on Saturday and Sunday. Because I might never see my home again and I had a substantial job ahead of me to get my affairs in order, I asked to come on Sunday so they could examine me on Monday. It was really only one working day difference and gave me four days at home to get straightened out. This new doctor stated that if I was not there "tomorrow," he would not treat me. Later I realized that it was not the one day that was important. It was being certain that I would make the commitment to do everything it would take to fight cancer and win.

A diagnosis of cancer is not a death sentence. Half of all patients, including those who give up, are saved. For some types of cancer, over 9 out of 10 people can be considered cured. Of the others, many go into remission or have their cancer controlled for a long period of time. Indeed, there are sunrises as well as sunsets to be enjoyed. See that they make plans for living with cancer and its treatments. See that they make plans for living.

Work with the patient, discuss, coerce, convince, do whatever is necessary so that the patient makes a true commitment to do everything in their power to fight their disease. It will save untold painful decisions later on with the possibility of many resulting mistakes. By doing everything automatically that could possibly be helpful, their life will be much easier and probably better.

Getting in Charge 3

Possibly the most common complaint is that the patient has given up. For one reason or another, they just refuse to do anything to help themself. Maybe the doctor has told them they are terminal. Maybe they have been told they are curable. The prognosis is not what seems to be the deciding factor. The supporter is frantic. She does not know what to do or how to get the patient to try to fight. She loves the patient and would do anything and has done everything.

And right there we generally have the cause of the problem. You love the patient; you would do anything for the patient, and you have done everything for the patient. What has happened with the best of intentions is that you have taken away all control from the patient.

You and others have talked with the doctors, you and others have planned the treatments, you and others have scheduled everything that needs being done, you and others do everything for the patient that the patient needs. This is not a question of intentions. There is no doubt that your intentions are the best. You love the patient and you want to show it by caring for them. But sit back and think about what kind of a message this is sending them.

By doing everything for them you are saying that they are not capable of doing it. You are saying that they are "sick." Your loved ones do not do these things for you. Why? Because they believe you are well. By your doing everything for them, they must believe that you believe they are in too bad a shape to do for themself. Possibly if the prognosis is good, you are sending a signal out that it is untrue. If it is bad, you are indicating that you agree. There is no hope.

You have taken their authority and responsibility away. They are a puppet to be manipulated by their medical team at your direction. They are unable to make decisions because they are denied the opportunity. Since they have no say, they have no reason to do anything. They are out of control. They have lost their reason for being, their will to live, their energy to fight.

So how do you correct the situation? It is difficult but not impossible. Put them back in charge. Stop doing for them that which they are capable of doing themself. Make them make the decisions that they can. Make them do for themself. They should read their own books, make their own phone calls, keep their own lists, schedule their own appointments, and do all their personal things that they are able and capable of doing themself and that, if they were healthy, they would normally be doing for themself. Treat them as a "person with cancer" rather than a patient, enabling them to maintain control and participate in their health care as opposed to being something health care is being done to.

Granted this is difficult. You want to show your love and caring. It is probably comparable to giving candy to an overweight baby. For the moment, it might seem like the proper thing to do to make the infant happy. In the long run, there is no doubt that the infant is far better off without the unneeded candy. Likewise, for the moment your doing everything might seem like the best or easiest way. In the long run, the patient is far better off, happier, and will appreciate your love and caring more by being allowed to do for themself.

Once they are back in control, you can determine a happy balance between your doing and their doing for themself. There are many ways you can show your devotion besides usurping their authority and control. Suggest, discuss, reason, even disagree. Like a child wants a parent to express authority, a patient wants an individual to display their concern and caring by actions other than that of being a servant.

You can help the seriously ill patient ward off feelings of helplessness and abandonment if you continue to share your activities, goals and dreams as before. Few of us who are well know what it is like to be placed in a position of dependency. Cancer strikes one's self concept as a whole person as well as threatening one's life. Feelings of helplessness are real enough when one is flat on one's back. Make every effort not to compound them by ignoring the wishes of the patient, or worse, by trying to make an invalid of a person who is up and around.

When I was in the hospital recovering from surgery, my wife would visit me all day and then drive back to the hotel room at night. I asked my doctor if I might walk her to the car and he gave me permission on the condition that I would not use the elevator. I had to walk down the two flights of steps and back up! He knew the value of getting me to do for myself, plus the exercise.

I got plenty of visits from my family, companionship with every meal, lots of back rubs and dozens of cards, but I had to make my own phone calls when I felt up to it, be in on all the discussions and decisions about my treatment and do whatever else I always did for myself.

Some patients do not want to accept help and burden their family and friends with such acts as child care, cooking, shopping, laundry and transportation. Convince them that you are doing this because you love them and you choose to do these things that they are incapable of doing at the present time. Reassure them that they can resume these acts when they are capable.

Friends and families are often most loving, supportive and caring when patients are weak and helpless. They begin to remove these rewards when the patient regains health. It is imperative that patients be encouraged to do what they can for themselves and receive love, support and affection for independence, not weakness. If all the rewards come from being weak, patients have a stake in illness and less incentive for getting well.

Five rules to accomplish this are:

1. Encourage patients to take care of themselves. Many family members rush in and take over with such comments as, "You're sick. You shouldn't be up and around like that." The family should comment instead on their loved one's strength: "I think it is great the way you are taking care of yourself."

2. Comment on progress. Observe signs of improvement and let the patient know how pleased you are.

3. Spend time with the patient in activities unrelated to the cancer. Having cancer does not require that you and the patient stop enjoying yourselves. On the contrary, the more enjoyable life is, the greater the incentive is to stay alive.

4. Continue to spend time with the patient as they get well. Offer continued attention and support during recovery.

5. Treat the patient as if you expect them to live. You need not believe they will recover; you need only believe they *can* recover. This is asking a great deal when families and patients have received all the societal programming that says cancer equals death. But your beliefs matter enormously. The ideal is to have a positive belief that the treatments are a strong and powerful ally and that the patient can get well.

Give them the gift of hope. Restrain yourself, even though it hurts. Let them make their own mistakes. Give them the gift of getting back in charge. Pulling one's own weight is good exercise.

Knowledge 4

It is easier to come to grips with the reality of any crisis if we replace ignorance with information. There is much to learn about each type of cancer, its treatments, the possibility for recovery and methods of rehabilitation. Individuals well-versed in facts are less likely to fall prey to old wives' tales, to quacks touting worthless cures or to depressing stories of something that happened years ago to someone else. The more you know, the less you have to fear.

Fighting cancer is not a simple matter of thinking positively, wishing it away and saying, "Hey, doc, cure me." It is a matter of knowledge. It is a matter of the patient educating themself about every detail and mustering all their resources. They must use every drop of energy in an organized fashion to constructively concentrate on getting rid of cancer. Most cancers can be successfully treated, but generally there is only one chance. If they miss that first chance, if they don't do everything in their power, often there is no second chance. This is why no cancer patient can afford the luxury of looking back and saying, "I wish I would have...." Never look back. Have them concentrate on this moment forward and do everything in their power. There is no downside risk. Now they may have a chance.

The next step you can take is to help them acquire knowledge. They, personally, must find out all they can about their disease. When they try, they will be amazed how simple and interesting it is, even with their lack of medical background.

First and foremost, they should talk to their personal doctor who diagnosed them. Be certain to tape record or write down all his answers. The patient is not a professional, and they will be confused and forget. You may offer to visit their doctor with them. In the stress of the moment, they might not hear or understand everything the doctor says or misinterpret what is said. After a while, they will be amazed at what they understand. And remember, this is their life. It isn't their doctor's, it isn't anyone else's. If they want help, they had better help themself first. Later they can count on others to assist them.

Help them find out what kind of cancer they are supposed to have. This would include type, stage, grade, location, size, spread, receptors, differentiation, virulence, types of treatment it is receptive to, types of treatment their doctor believes it is not receptive to, and anything else their doctor can tell them.

Telephone 1-800-4-CANCER or go to www.cancer.gov – this is the U.S. Government's Cancer Information Service – or the Bloch Cancer Hotline at 1-800-433-0464 or through our website at www.blochcancer.org. Everything we do is free. Ask for a PDQ (Physicians Data Query) state-of-the-art cancer treatment computer print-out for their type and stage of cancer. This will show them the recognized standard therapy for their specific disease. Next, ask for a PDQ computer printout of open protocols (organized clinical trials of experimental treatments) for their specific type and stage of cancer from the entire U.S. This will tell them briefly about every experimental therapy currently available for their disease. It will allow them to know that there are other options just in case their state-of-the-art therapy does not work.

From the Bloch Cancer Hotline, request a free copy of Fighting Cancer, which is a step-by-step guide of things a patient can do to help fight the disease along with their treatments. You or the patient can also call the Bloch Cancer Hotline (or do this online) to request to speak to a person who has had the same type of cancer and has beaten it. Also from the Bloch Cancer Hotline, ask for a list of institutions that provide qualified second opinions. All of this and much more is available for the asking.

Get accustomed to calling 1-800-4-CANCER for most things you want to know and be very specific in what you request. The wonderful people there are trying to help you, but they can't guess what you are thinking.

PDQ, written in understandable English, will give a great deal of up-to-the-minute information on their disease. It will tell them how it is staged and what the overall statistics on their specific stage are. Remember, however, the patient is not a statistic. If they make it, their chances are 100%; if they don't, they are 0%. There is no in-between.

Clinical trials (experimental therapies) are a wonderful thing. For purposes of discussion here, there are fundamentally two types of trials. First, there are trials for generally difficult types of cancer. The procedure is usually to start off with the state-of-the-art therapy. If that should fail, they are switched to the next line of defense. If that fails, they then go to the third line, etc. After all standard therapies have been exhausted, they go for experimental therapies. Clinical trials are undertaken when there is a strong possibility that the new approach will improve cancer treatment. Each clinical trial offers a chance to live. It should work in theory. Maybe it can work for them. They have nothing to lose.

The second type of trial is a randomized, or sometimes called a double blind trial. This is where there is a difference between two or three types of treatments or dosages or methods, and it is desired to find out which is better. Absolutely no one can say for sure that one is better than the other. Individuals are asked to volunteer where they have no real preference and receive one of the methods, possibly without even their knowledge of which they are receiving. Then the results are monitored to find out which is better. For example, half the participants might receive a dose each month and the other half might receive a 1/4 dose each week to see which group does better. Maybe half would receive their treatment in the morning and the other half in the afternoon. Either way, this is possibly helping patients in the future and in no way hurting the patient. Patients who participate in trials have the opportunity to receive the most advanced care available - either the new treatment or the best standard therapy. If the new treatment is successful, trial patients are the first to benefit, and they have the satisfaction of helping themselves and others.

Usually, the diagnosis of cancer is given by the patient's family doctor. It is important, at this time, to call in a board certified oncologist (a doctor who specializes only in the treatment of cancer). Talk to this doctor and get the same information. Again, be certain they write all answers. If the patient relates well to this qualified physician, and they believe he can successfully treat them, the patient should have complete faith in him and do everything recommended. Once they have found this doctor, they should stop looking for other physicians and use all their energy to get well.

If, however, they do not relate well to this doctor or do not have faith in him, or he does not believe they can be successfully treated, go for a true second opinion. Having their original doctor recommend another doctor is often like getting a second first opinion, not an independent second opinion. So this means leaving the comfort of their original doctor and hospital and going across the street or across the city to a different medical system. The best they can do for themself would be a "multidisciplinary second opinion." This is by one of the Comprehensive Cancer Centers or a major hospital you can find by calling 1-800-4-CANCER, the Bloch Cancer Hotline at 1-800-433-0464 or at www.blochcancer.org. These specialists will tell them everything about their disease and answer any questions they or their family have openly and honestly. They will hear all their options.

If they are unable to get a multidisciplinary second opinion, find a second oncologist totally away from their present doctor or hospital. Get the same information from him. If again you get the impression that this physician cannot successfully treat them, go further. Cancer is a disease in which the patient must be very selfish and think only of themself.

Using PDQ protocols, look up who is doing the most work in their type of cancer and have the patient call him on the telephone explaining

---

DEFINITIONS

CURE: No sign of cancer and statistically should not recur.

REMISSION: No sign of cancer but statistically might recur.

CONTROL: Growth rate reduced to where it is not life-threatening.

ARRESTED: Growth stopped (possibly temporarily, possibly permanently).

---

their problem. Ask straight out if he believes they can be successfully treated. Successfully treating them might not necessarily mean cure in their specific disease. It might be "control," it might be remission, it might be holding it where it is without getting worse. It is amazing how a qualified specialist can accomplish things a less skilled individual does not believe can be done. With the help of a computer or telephone, find the most skilled specialist who believes he can do the most for them and then go to him to be certain it is what they want. Then see that they place all their faith and efforts with this individual to help the physician accomplish what he has set out to do.

If you follow our suggestions, initially you did the most difficult single thing in the whole battle – you got them to make a commitment to do everything. Second, you got them to feel in charge. Third, you got them the best possible medical attention. Now it is time to rationally plan the rest of the actions necessary to complete their commitment. You want to see that they do everything and leave nothing out that could possibly help.

There is a saying that it takes six things to beat cancer. First is the best possible medical treatment. Second is the best possible medical treatment. Third, fourth and fifth are the best medical treatment. Sixth is a positive mental attitude. Without all six, they don't have a chance. But look at it in that perspective and relative importance. A positive mental attitude is not burying their head in the sand and saying, "I'm going to get well." It is doing everything within their power in addition to medicine to help themself recover.

That "everything" is to thoroughly read and digest the book *Fighting Cancer* that they received free from 1-800-433-0464 or www.blochcancer.org. It is written in layman's language to help them understand their disease and do everything in their power to help them fight it. The last chapter is a check list. Make absolutely certain that they have checked each item in the last chapter. Go over it question by question with them. This is for no one's benefit but their own. It is their life.

In order to be of maximum assistance to the patient, you should make every effort to learn as much as you can about all the factors that can influence their life and their thinking. Whenever serious illness is involved, one must consider all the possible medical treatments. Therefore, the better you understand all the ramifications of medical treatments, the better you are able to discuss this with the patient, explain truths and dispel myths, and try to help guide and assist them.

There are two schools of thought on patient education. One is for the patient not to know, to care or to worry. Years ago, doctors and family refrained from telling a patient they had cancer. In 1970, Annette's sister was operated on and sewn up without removing anything. Several months later she died from breast cancer without ever having been told what her disease was. The family knew but never told her. As a matter of fact, in those days, the word "cancer" was never mentioned by many. In Neil Simon's play, *Brighton Beach Memoirs*, he refers to "that disease" in a whisper.

The other school of thought is to explain

every aspect of the disease and treatment so the patient can understand and become an active participant, not a passive recipient. Today, oncologists are taught this latter method. It is believed the greatest resource to cure a patient is within the patient. There is a saying, "Doctors do not cure cancer. Patients cure themselves with the help of their doctor." The immune system kills the cancer with the help of the treatments.

There is an old tale with a great moral called the "wheelbarrow story." An individual carted scrap metal from machines in a plant to the junk pile hour after hour, day after day. The turnover in this position had been high, and the current employee was very slow and lethargic. The plant manager came to him one day and explained the entire process of producing their product and what an important place this individual had in continuously moving the scrap from the machine to the junk pile. He was an integral and vital cog in the entire operation. From that moment on, he did an outstanding job.

I believe the same thing applies in the recovery from cancer. If they can understand the part that they are able to perform, they can help themselves do an outstanding job in the successful treatment of their disease. It is for that reason that the following information on medical treatment is presented. It is so that you can understand what their options are, what their doctor is recommending, why it is being recommended, what it is intended to do and how it is supposed to do it. With you going over this information with them, it is hoped that their mind and their body will help the treatments do their intended job.

There are three types of treatments that must be considered in treating cancer. First are conventional medical treatments (such as surgery, chemotherapy, radiation and the other treatments described later in Part II) of which I am completely in favor when prescribed by a qualified physician and concurred with by an independent qualified second opinion. Conventional medical treatments always come first and foremost in treating cancer.

Second are termed complementary (such as prayer, relaxation, imagery and diet). They are methods of treatment that are used in addition to conventional medical treatments. I am completely in favor of any and all complementary forms of treatment as long as their physician says they will not specifically harm the patient or interfere with whatever medical treatments they are taking.

Third are alternative therapies, methods of treatment used instead of conventional medicine. These would include Laetrile, pure macrobiotic diets, Immuno-Augmentation Therapy (IAT), etc. I am totally and unequivocally opposed to any form of alternative treatments! Any alternative therapy that their physician says will not hurt and is done in addition to conventional treatments becomes complementary therapy.

Stay far, far away from alternative therapies because they can kill by denying access to the treatments that thousands of scientists have developed and perfected over the years. They must believe in and use every supplemental therapy that their physician says cannot hurt them. It is their life, and if they don't do everything possible to help themself, no one else will.

Sometimes you may hear a person describing a treatment as "unorthodox." In my opinion, that term should not be used. It merely indicates the person using it is unfamiliar with the treatment and is trying to discourage its use even though it might be helpful to the particular patient.

In the first half of the 20th century, anyone being cured from cancer would only have done so with surgery. Therefore, to most surgeons, any method of treatment other than surgery, such as radiation, chemotherapy, relaxation or prayer was unconventional. Today most cancer patients receive a combination of therapies which results in much better success rates.

The critical thing to differentiate between is alternative and complementary treatments. Use your head and you will have no problem figuring out which is which. Everything recommended in this book is complementary. It is in addition to whatever their qualified physician recommends.

Some people don't like the prospect of taking an unpleasant medical treatment. Perhaps some doctor told them there was nothing medically that could be done, and they failed to seek a second opinion. A human being will not be denied hope. They get oversold on a complementary therapy and use it to the exclusion of medical treatments. Then this complementary therapy becomes an alternative therapy. It goes from something wonderful, something that can help save their life to something terrible, something that can most certainly cost them their life.

A mention must be made of spontaneous remission to let you know that it could be a factor, even though highly unlikely. This is where the patient, without any curative medical treatments, becomes completely cancer free for no explainable reason. Maybe it comes from prayer. Maybe it comes from visual imagery. No one knows where it comes from. It is my belief that someone who has a strong desire to live and does everything in their power is more apt to have a spontaneous remission.

There are hundreds of documented cases of spontaneous remission over the years. But out of the millions of cases of cancer, it is extremely rare. For someone to forsake medical treatments and expect spontaneous remission is like someone buying a $1.00 lottery ticket and quitting their job because they expect to win the $40,000,000 jackpot.

There are numerous commonly used treatments for cancer, many of which could be successful if used individually, but often are proved more successful when used in combination. I personally had radiation therapy, chemotherapy, surgery, immunization therapy and a year of adjuvant chemotherapy in addition to psychotherapy. The cure rate for patients with advanced Hodgkin's disease was increased from 54% to 84% by giving combination chemotherapy in an alternating pattern, demonstrating the complexities within a single type of therapy. Several of the more common medical treatments are discussed in Part II.

We have all heard war stories about various treatments for cancer and how horrible they are. I had five of the more common treatments. Prior to that, I was told I was terminal, that nothing could be done and that there was no hope. I lived for five days without hope. I want to go on record as stating that any single minute without hope is worse than all the treatments I went through!

These horror stories were probably true in your parents' or grandparents' time. Today, these treatments, when administered by qualified professionals, are scientific, not guess work. Doctors know exactly how much of anything can be given to you safely to do exactly what is supposed to be done and probably what the side effects or residual effects will be. Newspapers write up and show pictures of horrible fatal car accidents but rarely mention the hundreds of daily fender benders. With cancer, we hear about those who had severe problems but rarely about the many who had minimal problems.

By far, the greatest progress in cancer treatments has been made in recent years. Many cancers once thought to be untreatable are not only treatable but continue to increase in survival rates by using current therapies. At an annual review meeting of the National Cancer Advisory Board, Dr. Alan Rabson, when he was director of the Division of Cancer Biology and Diagnosis, referring to scientific highlights and discoveries, stated, "It has been one of the most exciting years during my lifetime." Dr. Lloyd Old of Memorial

Sloan-Kettering, one of the most respected cancer specialists in the U.S., said that there had been more progress made in the cancer field in the last several months than in the previous 25 years he had been in research. Dr. Vincent T. DeVita, Jr., former director of the National Cancer Institute, stated, "The pace at which science is moving is so exciting that the fear is not being able to keep up between the laboratory and the clinic."

People were burned with radiation therapy years ago. Today, this should not happen. In the past, some people were poisoned with drugs. My recollection is that in an article some years ago in the *Washington Post*, the reporter was able to locate some six drug-related deaths nationally. They showed a picture of an infant superimposed over her death certificate stating this child was killed by drugs. What dramatic journalism! These six deaths were out of some 200,000 people who received chemotherapy that year. If you compare the risk to the reward, there is no comparison. In my opinion, that article, by frightening people away from the proper treatment, killed more people than drugs would for many, many years.

Some 40 years ago a radical mastectomy was the treatment of choice for breast cancer. Now it is rarely an option. Relatively no one should die from testicular cancer today. Many say the greatest advances have been made in childhood cancers.

Be grateful that dedicated doctors and scientists discovered the treatments and perfected them so today's patients are able to receive the benefits of them. Only a few years ago this was not possible. Because many people died previously, maybe your patient has a chance of beating cancer. Have them do everything their qualified doctor recommends to help save their life.

Sometimes it is difficult to convince the patient that they are recovering when they feel absolutely rotten. It is hard to be optimistic when they feel worse now than at the time of diagnosis. The schedule of radiation or drug treatments may seem endless. They are convinced that there never was a day when they did not feel awful; there never will be one when they will feel normal, if only they could remember how normal feels. Some even interpret these physical reactions to treatments as signs that the cancer is returning. This is rarely the case although it will be necessary to be reminded of this over and over.

You can try to change their depression to optimism by explaining that the name of the game is not to take treatments. It is to beat cancer.

If the treatments are making their big body feel so rotten, think of what they are doing to those weak, little cancer cells.

Articles in local publications or local media announcing gigantic breakthroughs in cancer should be viewed with skepticism and not allowed to raise false hopes or doubts. Generally, these can be checked out easily by calling 1-800-4-CANCER, the Cancer Information Service at the National Cancer Institute. Major breakthroughs, if publicly announced, would be important enough to make all the major wire services. You would hear about them on all the radio and TV news programs as well as in newspapers and magazines.

The following is from an article in *Good Housekeeping* by Dr. Alan E. Nourse about what you can do to avoid being taken in by cancer quackery.

"First, I think it is important to recognize what really is being done by modern medical science, slow as the progress may appear. Researchers are piecing together an immensely complicated puzzle, and progress is slow precisely because the puzzle is so intricate. To discover why a normal cell goes wrong and how to stop the process, we have to understand some of the most basic processes of life itself. But bit by bit the answers are coming in.

"Second, we should bear in mind that even though a 'magic bullet' against cancer may not be found, more and more kinds of cancer are being cured, and the list of known, effective treatments is lengthening.

"Third, knowing what we do about the dedication and integrity of most medical scientists, we should be suspicious of anyone who claims that researchers are deliberately hiding valid cancer cures from the public.

"But most important of all, we should use some plain good judgment. When you hear about a new cancer remedy that sounds simple and easy and that you can handle largely by yourself, recognize it for what it is. If it sounds too good to be true, it almost certainly *isn't* true."

Considering the Prognosis 6

There are very few of us who would give up a chance to look into an accurate crystal ball if we had the opportunity, even though we realize full well that we may not like what we see. It may hurt us. It may depress us. It may scare us. It may diminish our quality of life. But still we would look if we could.

Similarly, there are very few cancer patients who would not ask their physician what their prognosis (medical future) is. And why not? We are talking about a life-threatening disease. To fail to ask the question would imply that the patient feels there is no hope or that the patient thinks their physician feels there is no hope. If the doctor felt it were minor or could readily be successfully treated, he would certainly have volunteered the information. By not even asking their prognosis, the patient brings on doom and gloom.

Most patients, family members and friends find ways to deal with the reality of illness and the possibility of death, even when it involves themselves or their loved ones. They find the strength to bounce back from situations that seem to cause unbearable grief. Life is very short for everyone. Since there are no guarantees, we should make the most of each day.

It is important that the patient know the complete truth in every detail of the diagnosis. The patient, family and friends usually learn the diagnosis sooner or later. Most people find it easier for all if everybody can share their feelings instead of hiding them. This frees people to offer each other support. Patients agree that hiding the diagnosis from them robs them of their right to make important choices about their life and their treatments. Keeping the diagnosis secret denies loved ones the chance to express love and to offer help and support.

Family and friends also bear great emotional burdens and should be able to share them openly with each other and the patient. Even children should be told, as they sense when something is amiss and may imagine a situation worse than it really is. By sharing the diagnosis, patient, family and friends build foundations of mutual trust and understanding.

There is no such thing as a bad question. There are only bad answers. Asking the question brings on a whole array of possibilities. Remember, this book is being written to help you in supporting a cancer patient. Their problem can be anywhere from a pre-malignant condition that is theoretically

100% curable to a wildly metastasizing systemic disease with only a 2% chance for recovery. This extreme variance is magnified geometrically by the inherent characteristics of not one but two distinct individuals.

The first is the characteristics of the physician. He may be qualified and know about the up-to-the-minute state-of-the-art therapy for this particular type and stage of cancer, or he may be living in the antiquated world of last year or last decade. He may be trying to play God and demonstrate his importance and knowledge, belittling anyone else's potential role in helping. He may be of the old school and not believe in being completely honest with the patient. He may have gotten up on the wrong side of the bed, had an argument with his wife, be worried about a malpractice suit or thinking about the golf game he is missing. In other words, maybe his prognosis to the same patient the day before or the day after would have come out completely differently. And maybe the prognosis by a more experienced expert in this particular type and stage of cancer could present a far more accurate picture.

Second comes the variability in patients. Maybe the patient is in generally good health or bad. Maybe they are 29 or 92. Maybe they are truly happy, feel loved and needed, useful and productive, or maybe they have no reason to try to recover. Maybe they are going to keep all their doctor's appointments on time, take all their treatments as recommended, eat a well-balanced diet, seek support, say prayers, practice relaxation and visual imagery and do all the other things they can to help themself fight the disease.

At most, all a physician can do is tell a patient about the statistics of their disease. If you took 1,000 patients with this particular type and stage of cancer, "x%" would be cured. But this patient is not a statistic. They are not 1,000 patients. There is no possibility that they will end up "x%" cured. If they make it, their chances are 100%. If they don't, their chances are 0%. There is no in-between. Furthermore, any statistics are for patients getting this cancer and starting treatments at least five years before this time. Possibly as much as half of the progress in cancer treatments has come in the past five years. And maybe this patient caught their cancer earlier, is using better medical assistance, is doing more things right and has a stronger will to live.

I have even heard some ridiculous forecasts such as, "You have three years to live, and there is nothing that can help you." Who in the world knows what is going to be discovered next week or next month to say nothing of next year. If the person is going to die this afternoon or tomorrow or even later this week, they are probably terminal. But stating three months or three years is just a physician saying that he personally is unaware of what is possible or could be done. After all, I was given three months to live in 1978 with "nothing else that could be done."

And this brings around another philosophical line of thinking. We are all terminal and knew this from the time we were born. No one ever gets out of this world alive. One hundred years from now, we are all going to be together. Therefore, the problem is not to keep from dying. That's impossible. The problem is to delay dying as long as possible while maintaining the maximum quality of life. Quality of life is every bit as important as quantity.

Quality of life should be considered in two distinct aspects: the physical side and the emotional side. Both sides are equally important..

The physical side of the quality of life for a cancer patient must first concern itself with an absence of pain and suffering. Dr. Vincent T. DeVita, Jr., former director of the National Cancer Institute, stated, "Only 20% to 30% of cancer patients get severe pain; the rest don't. For those patients who have pain, there are plenty of drugs on the market to cover almost every kind of pain."

Next would be to examine the effects of treatments. There are so many myths about the horrors of cancer treatments that I have heard people say a painful death would be preferable to treatments. They know not what they say.

As explained in Part II, many of the current therapies have little or no side effects. The fact that they did years ago is of no consequence today. Great advances have been made in reducing the side effects of treatments. Further, the patient should adopt the attitude that the idea is not to take treatments but to defeat cancer. With this feeling, any side effects are welcomed rather than dreaded with the idea that they are fighting the disease.

This brings us around to the emotional side of the quality of life. The dominant factor is that it is much better to fight to live than wait to die. A physician completely ignores this fact when he arbitrarily recommends nothing or palliative therapy with the idea that the patient is too old or the statistics are too poor and it would hurt their quality of life. Nothing can hurt it worse than doing nothing. The patient should have the right to choose.

It is a foregone conclusion that the patient will and should ask their physician for a prognosis. The quantity and quality of their future must be the most important factor on their mind. Don't expect, encourage or accept a one word answer. Ask for a detailed explanation and question any aspects that appear unclear or incomplete. Don't elicit positive guarantees or possible outcomes. Seek only his ideas of what can be expected for this specific patient with this specific problem. Reduce it to writing at the time it is given along with all options.

Giving a cancer patient a reason for being is the field in which a friend or relative can excel. You have examined the feelings of a cancer patient. You have helped them make the commitment to fight and get in charge. You have helped them get knowledge and you have reviewed the ramifications of medical treatments. You have worked through the prognosis and realize that the quality of life in its truest sense is the most important factor. Now you can focus on helping in the fight against depression.

Cancer is an extremely depressing disease. The effect of malignant cells on our body is depressing. The diagnosis is depressing. The treatments are depressing. Realistically facing our own mortality is depressing. Being treated "differently" by friends because of cancer is depressing. Everything about this disease is depressing. Expect it, face it, know it will happen. Explain to the patient that it is normal to have this feeling. The idea is not to try to eliminate it but to minimize it and replace it with pleasant events so as not to dwell on the depression.

With most cancer patients, when getting under the surface feelings, depression is a paramount problem. It is perhaps the greatest single factor in the deterioration of their quality of life for most cancer patients. If it is allowed to continue, depression will grow until it becomes all consuming. Every human being is different and responds to different stimuli. Your goal is to experiment and find out what your patient reacts favorably to.

To say to a cancer patient, "Don't be depressed" is as foolish as telling Niagara Falls to stop running. As a matter of fact, it would possibly hurt the patient because it would focus their attention even more on their depression. What you must do is not try to convince them not to be depressed but to focus their attention on something they like so they will concentrate on that and forget their depression.

First, make them feel important. Make them feel truly needed. Give them a reason for being. Make them do the things they have always done and which they are still capable of doing. Let them make their decisions and some of yours, too. Let them decide what they want for lunch or dinner, what time they should turn in and even what you should wear when you go out. If they have been handling finances, certainly see that they continue if they are capable. Have them write their own notes and make their own phone calls. If they are not capable of writing, have them dictate to you. Let it be their act.

Next, plan things for the future. Set goals and plan things that will excite them and give them anticipation and joy thinking about from now until the time comes. Maybe it is a trip to somewhere they have always wanted to go. By planning it three or six months from now, they can have time to dream, study the maps, read up on what is happening there, talk to people about various aspects of the trip, and generally have three to six months of wonderful thoughts to help replace the depression that is inevitably present.

Maybe the event to plan could be as simple as renting a movie. After my surgery, the big occasion that I anticipated for three weeks was my first venture out to dinner and away from hospital food. I chose to go to Victoria Station for Prime Rib. The realization was nothing compared to the anticipation. But that doesn't make any difference at all. I now realize that for the three weeks of recuperation, I had the anticipation to distract me from my sorrows.

The event could be giving a party, simply being invited to a party, going on a picnic, a sleigh ride, a balloon ride, to the office, taking the kids to the zoo, playing cards with friends, a drive in the country or any action that would be pleasant to the patient. Whatever would conjure up visions of happiness will fit the bill. Provide a pedicure, manicure or hair stylist – anything to build their self-esteem. An act as simple as a massage or a foot rub can do the trick. Getting their thoughts away from depression or feeling sorry for themself to something more pleasant is the entire idea. Make an effort and you can do it.

Responsible pursuits keep life meaningful, and recreation keeps it zesty. Activities that give a sense of purpose and those that give enjoyment are necessary. Some people find that cancer is a spur to do fun, adventurous or zany things they've always wanted to do but have put off as being not quite responsible. This is good because it helps ward off two overreactions: one is giving up, and the other is trying to cram a life's worth of responsible accomplishments into a very short time.

There is no scientific or medical proof for it, but cancer patients who have "places to go and things to do" seem to live longer and feel better. "I'm too busy to schedule my demise, or maybe I just don't have the sense to lie down and let it happen." Many have found that they cannot retire from living. You just go through one day at a time and give it your best.

"Doing" is not the same as overdoing. Try to recognize limitations as well as capabilities. Fatigue can bring on crushing despair and many people have found that a safeguard as simple as adequate rest fends off depression. Exhaustion weakens our physical and emotional defenses. Pain also can make a mockery of attempts to function normally. Physicians are learning much about controlling pain without drugging the patient, so pain, especially if it is prolonged, should be discussed with the physician.

"Putting one's house in order" is a desire that strikes many who learn they have cancer. This is not the same as giving up. In fact, everyone needs to review their insurance policies, update wills and clean out the closets and drawers from time to time. It gives something constructive to do and relieves the stress of knowing it is undone.

Play is not an elective for health; it is essential. Play is any activity producing emotions of joy or the experience we call "having fun." Play forces us to change our perspective, suspend our limits, make up our own rules and then change them. Play requires creativity.

Creativity is particularly important when dealing with a disease considered "incurable." To conquer such an illness we must become creative, for if we accept the "expected" course of the illness, we will not get well. Play not only increases our energy but also enhances our will to live. Play improves the quality of life and makes it richer. It knocks us out of despair and increases our wish to live. In doing this, it supplies the energy needed in mustering the will to live.

Our society lays such great stress on the puritan work ethic that we adults must re-learn how to play. Because we may unknowingly apply our work attitudes to play, honest examination may sadly disclose that we are not really enjoying our play time. Make a list of 20 playful activities for the patient. Relabel their play time as work. Schedule play time and see that they honor it as being equally important as work time. As it is possible to overwork, it is possible to overplay. Strike a balance between these two equally important aspects of a full and healthy life.

One of the major things you need to do is to listen carefully to the patient and clarify exactly what they are "really" saying. How are they "really" feeling? How can you "really" be helpful? If they are angry and annoyed about little things, is it because they had a bad day at the office, because of concern over a new symptom or because they got up on the wrong side of the bed? You must clarify the source of the irritation before deciding to sympathize, suggest seeing a doctor or ignore the mood. Do not rush in to propose a solution to a problem before being certain of what the problem "really" is. Recognize the difference between complaining that relieves stress and complaining that reinforces and festers negative stress.

It is vitally important to have good communication between the support person and the patient. Failing to do this could cause a wall to build up, increasing unwanted stress on both sides. Make it a point to open up a dialogue between family and patient to be able to talk about things in depth. Share your feelings openly. It will help both parties and will lead to meaningful discussions.

Suggesting Actions 8

The phrase, "I'd like to help, but I don't know what I can do" can no longer be a part of your vocabulary. In this one chapter we shall try to go through a multitude of specific actions you can take to assist a cancer patient over and above conventional medical treatments. Not one of them includes the words, "I'm sorry." Every single one of them contains actions to imply that you care and you are with them every step of the way to help fight this disease.

While all kinds of actions are important, I would rate at the top getting the patient to practice relaxation and visual imagery 3 times a day for 15 minutes each. It has powerful potential to help and no possibility of hurting if done properly. Some time ago, when there were only 3,000 board certified medical oncologists, there were 5,000 individuals trained and professionally teaching relaxation and visual imagery. It is never recommended in lieu of medical treatments. Only in addition to them.

Two cancer treatment specialists rationalized that if the mind played a function in causing cancer, as many people believe, why couldn't the mind be trained to help treat the cancer. They started a clinic in 1976 and brought 150 cancer patients there. These were not normal cancer patients, though. They had two unique qualities. First, they were terminal because their doctor said they were going to die imminently from their cancer. Second, they could have no possible medical treatments such as chemotherapy, surgery, radiation, hyperthermia, immunotherapy, etc. These people were going to die from their cancer.

They taught these people two things. First of all, they taught these people to relax. Not just superficially, but a way down deep relaxation. It is a scientifically proven fact that tumors grow faster in mice under stress. What is the dangerous part about cancer? The fact that it will continue to grow! If it never grew from where it is, the patient could live another 100 years with it. If, by relaxing, the growth rate of the tumor could be slowed, there is no question they would be better off.

Second, the specialists taught these people to visualize their cancer and think it away. Sound silly? Some two years later, when Annette and I read about them in the newspaper, of the initial group of 150 terminal cancer patients using only their minds to think away the cancer, some 10% were completely free of cancer. Another approximately 10% were dramatically improved. A third roughly 10% had their cancer stabilized.

My wife and I made up our minds that if this gave me a 30% chance of staying alive instead of none, we were going to go there. As it was, the doctors felt they could successfully treat me. However, I used relaxation and imagery in conjunction with the medical treatments. I cannot say that it is what cured me, but I can state without any question that it made me feel better. I believe it helped, and I positively know it did not hurt me. I would never recommend this in lieu of medicine but only in addition to everything else the physician wants to do.

For a graphic demonstration of what visual imagery is, close your eyes and imagine you are holding a fresh yellow lemon in your left hand. Pretend to take a knife in your right hand and cut the end of the lemon off. Imagine holding the rest of the lemon above your mouth, sticking your tongue out and squeezing lemon juice on your tongue. What happens? You start to salivate. You cannot help yourself. Absolutely nothing happened except that you imagined lemon juice dripping on your tongue, and your saliva glands started working. It is the same theory that, by imaging your thymus gland, you are able to increase the production and flow of natural killer cells and maybe they are able to control or destroy malignant cells.

Some children successfully employ the use of visualization by imagining their natural killer cells looking like Pac-Man gobbling up their cancer bit by bit. One researcher at a prestigious mid-western institution was able to induce complete remission in two children with terminal brain cancer after all medical treatment had failed.

There is no right way and no wrong way to do these exercises. The only important thing is to do them regularly. A patient is not supposed to feel anything at the time. This could be compared to radiation therapy, where the patient feels nothing when the treatment is given. Several recommended methods of practicing relaxation and visual imagery are explained in the book Fighting Cancer, available free by calling 1-800-433-0464 or through www.blochcancer.org.

CDs to help understand and practice relaxation are available from numerous sources including private practitioners and public libraries. If you have a problem finding one locally, you may request one free by calling the Bloch Cancer Hotline at 1-800-433-0464 or locally 816-854-5050. You also can hear it on our website at www.blochcancer.org.

As a supporter of a cancer patient, you would

be wise in personally practicing the relaxation part of the exercise regularly, at least twice a day. You are naturally under a great deal of stress and the more you can control it and remain calm and serene, the better it is for you and the more you can help the patient. By practicing relaxation twice a day, you will find yourself much more tolerant and easy going. You will be able to do a great deal more for the patient without becoming irritable, impatient and stressed out. Try it for ten days. You'll notice a big difference.

A simple action can mean a great difference in results. If I were to buy a building that required a great deal of money to fix up, I would like to know it had a good foundation so that my efforts would not be in vain. The same concept applies to a cancer patient. Before spending a lot of time taking treatments and possibly expending their one chance to beat the disease, make certain their attitude is receptive to winning. See that the patient takes the mental attitude quiz in the book *Fighting Cancer* or available free by calling the Bloch Cancer Hotline at 1-800-433-0464 or locally 816-854-5050 and requesting "Quiz." The "Quiz" is also on our website at www.blochcancer.org.

This test has not been proven scientifically accurate and is certainly not meant to change any attitudes. It is only meant to find out the patient's deep down feelings on how anxious they are to recover and how much they are willing to do to accomplish this. If the quiz shows their attitude is good, go for it. If not, wouldn't it be wise to seek competent counseling to try to correct the situation as early as possible?

Try to get the patient to join a support group. There are many psychologists who believe this is extremely important in the patient's scheme of recovery. In a Stanford University study, a specific group of patients who attended weekly support group sessions survived almost twice as long as patients receiving just routine cancer care. Support groups range from organizations like the Cancer Support Community with locations across the U.S. and online at www.thewellnesscommunity.org, the American Cancer Society, and many cancer specific organizations with their weekly, professionally supervised support groups and numerous daily programs, to church groups that meet monthly or twice a month.

Like everything else, often it is difficult to get the patient to start. It is foreign to the way we have been raised. We are taught not to discuss our problems with others. Once they break the ice and get comfortable, they will find it among their better times. Having spent a great deal of time at numerous support programs, it appears to substantially help the quality of life of participants. If there is one available for supporters of cancer patients, get yourself involved in it. You, too, can benefit.

To find out where there are support groups in your area, call places like the American Cancer Society, the Leukemia Society, a cancer-specific hot line, a church or mental health agency, local hospitals or look in the newspaper under support programs. Something should be available if you try. If you live in a very remote area that is too far to commute to the nearest town, see if you can locate neighbors who have had a similar problem who would be willing to get together possibly weekly to discuss whatever they have on their minds. If each patient brings one or two supporters, it only takes three or four patients plus their supporters to have a nice group. Many cancer specific organizations have online support groups for those unable to attend a support group.

Get the patient to laugh at every opportunity and create those opportunities often. See that they watch humorous television programs, listen to funny radio shows, attend humorous movies or go to comic stage shows. It is easy to rent old Laurel & Hardy, the Three Stooges or Marx

Brothers films and show them at home or in a hospital room. Norman Cousins claimed he healed himself with humor. It certainly can't hurt, and it makes most people forget their problems and feel better.

Getting the patient a pet can do wonders. Having a little puppy or a cat to care for, to talk to, to pet, to feed and just to smile at can improve the quality of life. If a pet is out of the question, a plant can provide many of the same benefits with a much smaller degree of responsibility.

Another way you can assist a cancer patient is with their plan of physical activities. All oncologists I have heard recommend exercise within reason. It is beneficial both physically and emotionally. The theory is to do as much as they can in view of their background, their specific problems and their physical condition, but not to overdo exercise. Therefore, there is no pat rule applicable to all patients.

One individual recovering from serious surgery may be doing well to lift their arm 45 degrees 3 times a day while another could do their normal time on an aerobic circuit. If the patient is capable but has not been used to exercising, you should assist them. Play a game with them. Go for a walk with them at their pace for whatever time is reasonable. Do not let them vegetate. Do whatever you can with them to keep them moving as long as you do not overtire them.

Another area in which you can assist is diet and nutrition. This is an extremely complex area with a great many assumptions and very few probable facts. Everyone's taste is different and further affected by the treatments they may be receiving, as well as their image of their weight and what they would like it to be. With that in mind, let's see if we can come up with some generalizations.

There is a saying that if a person is going to recover from cancer, it is going to be their own immune system that cures them with the help of their doctors. Since the strength of the immune system is directly proportional to nutrition intake, it is vital that the patient eats a well-balanced diet sufficient to maintain their strength. This is further compounded by the fact that many treatments hinder a person's desire or ability to eat. Therefore, a concentrated effort is required to consume a well-balanced diet.

This is no time to go on any fad diets or try to lose weight. Certain cancers are evidenced by a loss in weight; so, it is that much more important to maintain weight. High fiber, low fat diets may or may not help in preventing cancer. The jury is still out. But there is no place for it in fighting cancer.

Macrobiotic diets or any other kind of unbalanced diet may be touted on the same grounds that any medicine that tastes bad enough must be good for you. However, there is no evidence that they will help your immune system. As a matter of fact, most professional dieticians state that a well-balanced diet is the best for enhancing the immune system.

Take your patient out to restaurants that serve well-balanced meals, not just fast food places. Fix them healthy, varied meals at home even though they ask for a very limited menu. Urge them to eat a sufficient quantity, even if it means forcing themself. An attractively prepared dish can be much more appealing and possibly enhance their desire to eat. Play games to get them to eat like you would with a baby. They need your help and you can demonstrate your love and caring by taking your time and patience to get them to eat enough well-balanced foods.

While they are eating enough, they should keep themself active in whatever projects are normal in their lives that they can continue. If they work or go to school and they are capable of continuing while on treatments, they certainly should. If they have to reduce their activities slightly and that is possible, they should. If they have to take a few days off during treatments, they should and then go back and resume. If they cannot maintain their pre-cancer lifestyle, find something less strenuous that they enjoy and get them into it. If they can't continue to be a gym instructor, maybe they can teach English.

If they can't appear seven nights a week in a road company, maybe they can sing in a church choir. Maybe they can do part time work for a hospital or other charitable organizations.

Put your mind to it and you will see that there are many options. The easy thing for them to do is sit back and do nothing, but that is the least healthy. Find something constructive to keep their mind and body occupied. There is a saying, "Idle hands get into mischief." Idle minds will conjure up all kinds of bad things and allow the patient to concentrate on negatives without hope for relief. Keeping mentally occupied will minimize depression and allow them to think pleasant thoughts.

The days can be more valuable if they can learn to enjoy mundane moments as well as memorable occasions. This is true whether they have weeks or years left. It is true, in fact, whether they have a life-threatening disease or not. Physical well-being is closely tied to emotional well-being. The time the patient takes in not dwelling on their cancer strengthens them for the time they must devote to fighting it.

Another field of assistance, apparently regardless of a person's beliefs, can be prayer. A trial was done at the University of California-San Francisco with patients for open heart surgery. They were randomized into a trial group and a control group by a computer so that both groups were identical. No one knew who was in which group. The patients, the doctors and the nurses did not know. No one knew. The names of the patients in the trial group were given to students at a monastery to pray for several times a day. After the trial was over, the results were analyzed. The patients in the trial group had a significantly faster recovery with fewer side effects.

The implications of that are mind boggling to me. Imagine how the results could have been enhanced if the doctors and nurses knew who was being prayed for, to say nothing of the patients themselves. When I was going through treatments, a friend advised he was saying a prayer for me every day. I told my wife I had to get well to fulfill his prayers. It made me feel so great.

No matter what your beliefs or those of the patient, say prayers for them and let them know you are saying prayers for them. Try your best to get them to say prayers for themselves. Maybe no one can prove that it will help, but there is no possible way it could hurt. If it did nothing but keep their mind occupied that much longer, it would improve the quality of their life. In all probability, it can do a lot more than that.

Touching, holding and hugging are ways to express the acceptance and caring that is so important to the patient. More than words, they show love and express your belief in the patient's continued desirability as a physical being. Disfigurement or debilitation caused by treatment can affect reactions. Look beyond these physical changes to the person within, the one who more than ever needs your love and physical reassurance of that love.

Admittedly, it is a difficult time. Beset by treatment reactions, anxiety, self-doubt or possibly by a mistaken notion of what your feelings are might cause the patient to withdraw from you. Try to prevent a cycle of misunderstanding from developing. As the well partner, try to feel sure in your love and reach out gently and repeatedly, if necessary, to provide the reassurance that cancer cannot destroy your relationship. Talk openly with tact and restraint about the patient's physical appearance and your understanding and continued devotion to them.

Summary 9

With all your concern for the patient, do not forget to take care of yourself. If you allow yourself to get overly tired, run down and ill, you will not only be of no possible help, but possibly a hindrance. Instead of an asset, you could become a burden at least emotionally if not physically.

Pace yourself. Give yourself space. Limit your time spent with the patient and allow yourself time for outside activities. Get away by yourself or with others and clear your mind. In this way, you can actually do more for the patient in the long-run. Eat well. Sleep well. Take care of yourself.

It is wonderful to make the patient feel better, be happy and think highly of you for the moment. Your true goal is to have the patient recover and have the best quality of life possible. Consider each action on your part and its long range implications. Do everything you can that will help, and nothing that will hurt their chances of recovery and their long-term quality of life.

The following is a list of some suggestions for you to follow to be of maximum benefit to your patient:

→ Don't be afraid to use the word cancer. Call it what it is.

→ Make it clear that you are with the patient to help and give support, not to offer sympathy. Be calm and just be there.

→ Be a good listener.

→ If the patient expresses feelings of being a burden, reassure them by saying you have chosen freely to be there.

→ Treat the patient as if you expect them to live. You need not believe they **will**, you only need believe they **can** recover.

→ Have patience. Not everyone hears the information the first time.

→ Don't be afraid to cry with the patient and family. This can lead to meaningful conversations.

→ Don't tell them to keep a stiff upper lip or keep smiling. You can say it must be very hard or very tiring or very frightening.

→ Allow them to express anger when it is to relieve stress.

→ Express love, caring and concern verbally

and through actions at every opportunity. Letters, cards and flowers are tangible methods.

→ Cancer is not contagious. Touch, hug, kiss. Human contact is very necessary.

→ The patient needs reassurance that you love them even though their physical appearance might have changed.

→ Give them something special they might not want to buy for themself.

→ Provide companionship with the patient during meals and other appropriate times.

→ Act cheerful whenever you are around the patient. Being depressed and gloomy is contagious, and the patient could catch it.

→ Be completely honest with the patient in a constructive and optimistic manner.

→ Keep no secrets from the patient.

→ Do not whisper to others in front of the patient.

→ Think of the patient as an individual, a unique human being, not a statistic.

→ Discuss all the normal things with the patient that they have always been interested in. While cancer might have become the dominant item in their life, their interests have not changed.

➡ Encourage the patient to believe that their actions could make a difference in the outcome and the quality of their life.

➡ Make no prognosis. It can only cast doubts on your credibility.

➡ See that the patient makes a verbal commitment to do everything in their power to fight the disease.

➡ Allow the patient to make all his/her own decisions when possible.

➡ Encourage the patient to learn everything about their cancer that they can.

➡ Make them do everything for themself that they can. This includes making telephone calls, reading, keeping lists, scheduling appointments, and doing personal things.

➡ See that they treat their cancer promptly, properly and thoroughly.

➡ Make certain their doctor is qualified to treat them and believes he can successfully treat them.

➡ See that they relate well to their physician. Have them write down all their questions before seeing their physician and make sure they understand the answers.

➡ They should receive a PDQ computer printout from 1-800-4-CANCER, or www.cancer.gov, or by calling the Bloch Cancer Hotline at 1-800-433-0464 and make certain they are getting the state-of-the-art therapy.

→ Be certain they read, understand and practice everything in *Fighting Cancer*.

→ They should understand each component of their treatment as to what it is, what it is supposed to do and how it is supposed to do it.

→ If the patient has adverse side effects from treatments, encourage them to realize what it is doing to those weak cancer cells.

→ Keep pleasant activities planned for the future.

→ True love is never having to say, "I'm sorry." Erase that phrase from your vocabulary. Sympathize with them, not for them.

→ See that the patient spends 15 minutes, 3 times a day practicing relaxation and visual imagery.

→ Be certain the patient takes the mental attitude quiz in the book *Fighting Cancer*.

→ Get the patient into one or more support groups or set one up. Join one yourself if available.

➡ Plan regular physical exercise in accordance with their abilities.

➡ Advise the patient that you are saying prayers for them and urge them to say prayers for themself.

➡ Do not assume the patient is going to die. Many are cured.

➡ See that the patient eats a well-balanced diet sufficient to maintain their strength and their weight.

➡ A pet can be very beneficial in providing a purpose, companionship, pleasant tasks in caring, and amusement.

➡ Record messages, favorite music or books.

➡ Share your feelings with the children. Allow them to participate and help with the care. Help them talk and share their feelings.

➡ Encourage the patient to keep as physically and mentally active as they are capable.

➡ Don't be afraid to be funny and laugh. Laughter is therapy. Rent funny movies. Give joke books.

➡ Do not tell horror stories of other cancer patients.

➡ Talk about past occasions and reminisce

about good times. Discuss how they have been special and meaningful to your life.

→ Never discourage an optimistic outlook.

→ See that the patient keeps themself clean and neat at all times. Personal hygiene is very important.

→ Provide pedicure, manicure, hair stylist or pretty scarves – anything to build their self-esteem. Give a make-up lesson or gentle massage.

→ Encourage a second opinion.

→ See that they keep all appointments on time.

→ Do not encourage the patient to try alternative therapies.

→ As the patient gets better, do not diminish your attention to them. Subconsciously, they may wish themself ill only to regain your lost attention.

→ Take care of yourself.

Do everything you can as the opportunity presents itself so that you will never look back and say, "I wish I would have. . ." You did not create the problem. You did not cause the problem. You have no control over the outcome. Regardless of the results, if you care and do everything possible at the time, there can be no blame. You tried your best, and that is all any human being can do. With your help, the medical team's help and the patient's efforts, let's hope and pray that the outcome is every bit as good as can be desired.

What you just read are suggestions for you, the primary caregiver, to help the patient. The following are suggestions for you to help yourself so you can continue to be most effective for the patient:

1. Be considerate of yourself. Remember that you are a supporter, not a magician.

2. You cannot change anyone else. You can only change the way you relate to them.

3. Find a hermit spot. Use it daily.

4. Give support, encouragement and praise to friends and professionals. Learn to accept it in return.

5. At times you are bound to feel helpless. That is normal. Don't be hard on yourself.

6. Change your routine often and your tasks when you can.

7. Recognize the difference between complaining that relieves and complaining that reinforces negative stress.

8. Each night, focus on a good thing that happened during the day.

9. Be a resource to yourself.

10. If you never say "no," what is your "yes" worth?

11. Don't feel guilty when you take time off for yourself.

Winner vs. Loser

The Winner is always part of the answer.

The Loser is always part of the problem.

The Winner always has a program.

The Loser always has an excuse.

The Winner says, "Let me do it for you."

The Loser says, "That's not my job."

The Winner sees an answer for every problem.

The Loser sees a problem for every answer.

The Winner sees a green near every sand trap.

The Loser sees sand traps near every green.

The Winner says, "It may be difficult, but it is possible."

The Loser says, "It may be possible, but it is too difficult."

Be a Winner!

Part II   Cancer Treatments

SURGERY: At a meeting at the National Cancer Institute, we were told that surgery is given credit for 60% of those cured from cancer. Radiation therapy is credited for 25% and chemotherapy 15%. As you can see from these statistics, if someone has a tumor that is surgically removable, their case has an optimistic outlook.

But don't get the wrong impression. First of all, not too many years ago surgery was the *only* possible treatment for cancer. Therefore, surgery's current cure rate of 60% is a reduction from 100% a short time ago.

Secondly, don't confuse inoperable with incurable. Maybe they sound somewhat alike, but they don't mean anything similar. I was inoperable and here I am writing this book. Inoperable means that at the moment, in the opinion of the doctor who is examining you, it cannot be operated on. It does not mean that the patient cannot be successfully treated without surgery. Also, it does not mean that other treatments could not make the patient operable. In my case, radiation and chemotherapy reduced the size of the tumor to the point where it was operable. In addition, it does not necessarily mean that another surgeon with more experience or skills could not successfully perform the surgery.

Surgery, other than taking a biopsy or debulking a tumor, is generally used in cancer treatment only when it can cure a patient or solve a particular problem, such as a stopped-up colon or ureter. Therefore, other than for neuroendocrine cancers, surgery cannot be expected to completely cure a patient, it would not be considered the treatment of choice. Other options should be examined.

Furthermore, in my personal opinion, while surgery is properly given credit for 60% of those cured from cancer, I believe that failure to give additional treatments prior to or following surgery is responsible for many of the deaths from cancer. I was given radiation first to make my tumor operable, but I was also given a short course of chemotherapy prior to surgery so that my cancer would not metastasize during the period of time I was recuperating from the surgery. That is why I urge every patient to receive a multidisciplinary opinion prior to any treatment, or to confirm with a board-certified oncologist the surgeon's statement that no further treatments are necessary.

Some refuse surgery because of the fear that it will spread cancer. This should never be a concern. In the hands of a properly trained surgeon today, cancer cannot and will not be spread because of surgery.

Since surgery is the treatment of choice in many cancers, the National Cancer Institute is proposing to direct a major expenditure for improving the use of surgery in cancer cases. At the beginning of a presentation on improving surgery, we were given a note of caution in the form of a quotation from an eminent surgeon: "There must be a final limit to the development of manipulative surgery. The knife cannot always have fresh fields for conquest and although methods of practice may be modified and varied, and even improved to some extent; it must be within a certain limit, that this limit has nearly if not quite been reached. It will appear evident if we reflect on the great achievements of modern operative surgery; very little remains for the boldest to devise or the most dexterous to perform." This quote is from Sir John Erickson and was published in *Lancet*, a leading British medical publication on June 15, 1863!

CHEMOTHERAPY: Once the black sheep of cancer treatments, chemotherapy has become the leading weapon for increasing the number of patients who can be cured of cancer. At the same time, researchers are reducing the debilitating side effects that chemotherapy patients have typically had to endure.

"When chemotherapy was developed in the 1950s, cancer statistics were pretty much static," observed Dr. Bruce Chabner, former head of the National Cancer Institute's Division of Cancer Treatment. "Surgery had gone as far as it could go in curing local disease, and the radiation therapy of the 1960s and 1970s only improved the cure of local and regional disease.

"Unfortunately, at the time of diagnosis, about half of cancer patients already have spread of their disease beyond their original site, and the only therapy that has made inroads against these cancers is chemotherapy."

Now hundreds of thousands of patients with cancer who cannot be cured by surgery or radiation are being saved each year by drug treatments. As late as the 1980s, chemotherapy cured just a few thousand patients annually. Discoveries of ways to improve the effectiveness of drugs and overcome resistance to them, as well as better understanding of how cancer cells spread to other parts of the body, have produced new treatment tactics that should further increase drug cures and extend chemotherapy to common cancers not currently vulnerable to its effect.

"The prognosis for patients with disseminated malignancy has improved considerably," Dr. Chabner said. Especially notable is the increase in long-term disease-free survival time for patients with testicular cancer from 10% in 1973 to 96% in 2007. Similarly, the response rate for patients with ovarian cancer, stages I and II rose from 30% in 1973 to 92% (for stage I) and 85% (for stage II) in 2007. Further improvements in the efficacy of chemotherapy are expected to be attained with the refinement of high-dose chemotherapy, regional chemotherapy, bone marrow transplantation, the use of colony-forming assays to predict response, the use of combinations of genetically developed drugs, and the development of targeted therapies.

The new chemotherapy approaches are increasing the damage done to cancer cells and diminishing effects on normal tissue. Oncologists are also better able to control the occasional side effects of nausea and vomiting. Currently, few patients experience any nausea at all.

The importance of drugs is universally acknowledged now that cancer specialists realize that the disease is often systemic, or body-wide, not confined to one site or tissue. In such cases, only treatments like drugs that can reach the nooks and crannies of the body wherever cancer cells may be hiding can be successful.

Cancer cells lose their ability to control their own growth. Normal cells know when to stop growing. If half of your liver is removed in an operation, for example, your liver will grow back. Once local repair is complete, growth stops.

Something happens to cancer cells so that they lose their ability to respond to the body's signal to stop growing. Instead, they become wild, erratic cells that keep multiplying.

By themselves, cancer cells are not usually destructive, but they keep proliferating in the body so that they eventually crowd out the normal tissue of organs. That's what kills the patient. If the cancer is in the lungs, for example, the eventual replacement of healthy tissues by malignant cells interferes with breathing.

Many of the new drugs and biological agents now being tested are aimed at controlling the growth of cancer cells rather than destroying them. In a sense, we want to give cancer cells the correct signal to stop growing and behave like normal cells. The drugs fall into several main categories:

Alkylating agents: The genetic material, or DNA, of a cell is made up of chemical molecules, called bases, that must be duplicated and precisely paired when the cell divides. Alkylating agents interfere with the orderly pairing process and prevent successful division, so the cell dies. Some prominent drugs in this family are Leukeran (chlorambucil), Cytoxan (cyclophosphamide) and Paraplatin (carboplatin).

Nitrosoureas: This group of alkylating agents can cross the blood-brain barrier and get into the brain, unlike many other chemotherapy drugs. One such drug is called Carmustine, and it has been put into a wafer (Gliadel) used to treat certain types of brain tumors.

Anti-Tumor Antibiotics: These antibiotics do not act like the antibiotics used to treat infections. They are made from micro-organisms and they work throughout the time a cell is dividing. They prevent the strands of DNA from reforming after they are copied. They also block the cell's ability to make DNA. Adriamycin (doxorubicin) and bleomycin are two leading antibiotics in this category.

Antimetabolites: These drugs resemble nutrients that the cell uses to make DNA or other proteins needed by the cell. When these chemicals find their way into normal cell structures, they disrupt normal activity and the cell dies. Among these drugs are 5-FU (fluorouracil), 6-mercaptopurine (6-MP), fludarabine, cytarabine (Ara-C), and methotrexate (MTX).

Steroids: Steroids are used in cancer care because they change the way chemicals can get in and out of the cell. They also change how our body uses energy, how we store fluid and salt. Often, steroids are used with other medication. In that case, they may make the medication more effective, as in the situation where anti-nausea medicines are given with a steroid to make them more effective.

As more drugs are developed, categories change. Vinblastine and vincristine, derived from the periwinkle plant, prevent the cell from dividing. They, along with the drugs Taxol and Taxotere, are in the category called "Mitotic Inhibitors." The drug L-alparaginase and its newer cousin, Peg-L-asparaginase, are enzymes that destroy asparagine, an amino acid that some cancer cells can't make for themselves and must draw from the bloodstream. Normal cells, which synthesize the asparagine they need, are unaffected by the drug. These two drugs do not fall into a specific category.

Among the therapeutic changes that have taken place are:

• Adjuvant cancer therapy is now considered standard treatment. Adjuvant cancer therapy is giving chemotherapy and/or radiation therapy immediately after the tumor is removed by surgery. The drugs are believed to kill off the small amount of cancer cells that might still remain after the tumor was removed. This practice prevents metastasis and recurrence of the cancer.

- The use of "dose-dense" treatment regimens. This is an intensive drug regimen where each "cycle" is given closer together (every week to two weeks) and bigger doses of drugs are used. Dr. Chabner said, "We get the best results when patients are given full doses of the drugs as fast as possible immediately after surgery or radiation." Traditionally, when toxic effects of the drugs got too severe, doses would be lowered or the treatment stopped. Because of recently-developed medications to support the patient and prevent the blood counts from dropping dangerously low, patients are being successfully treated using the dose-dense method. This helps the patient tolerate the treatment, both physically and emotionally.

- The use of chemotherapy to shrink large tumors *prior* to surgery or radiation. This is called "neo-adjuvant" therapy. This technique shrinks some inoperable cancers into ones that can now be successfully removed with less time spent in the operating room or less radiation. This technique can also improve the cosmetic effects of cancer treatment, permitting less radical surgery or less extensive radiation.

- The development of analogues of established drugs that retain their cancer fighting properties but have fewer side effects. Abraxane is a drug that is made up of Taxol surrounded by a liposomal (fat) bubble. Although there is a high incidence of drug reactions to Taxol, there is less chance of reaction to Abraxane because the "fat bubble" surrounds the drug and protects the patient from contact with the drug. Eventually, the drug is very slowly released as the "fat bubbles" break down.

- The linking of toxic chemicals or radiation to monoclonal antibodies which only attack cancer cells. When the cell is attacked, the linked chemical is "delivered" to the cell. This technique, called regional perfusion, allows the medication to be delivered to the cancer cells, sparing the healthy cells.

- The discovery of new drugs that can overcome the resistance cancer cells often develop to established drugs. Drug resistance has been the major roadblock to the successful use of chemotherapy in patients with widespread metastatic disease. To overcome resistance, drugs are given in combination. Each drug attacks the cancer cells differently.

- Out of 1,000 laboratory-engineered chemical relatives of cisplatinum, the most potent chemotherapy agent, two have been found to retain their potency but have less severe side effects.

- More and more new biological therapies are being developed. In 2009, only ten new drugs were approved by the FDA. In 2010, sixteen new drugs were approved. In just the first four months of 2011, five new drugs had already been approved. Clinical trials can be found in most oncologists' offices and certainly at all major cancer centers.

- New biological therapies are being developed at a rate previously unheard of. In addition, it is possible to culture cells, examine the genetic components of the tumor, and choose a drug that will inhibit factors found within the tumor. This is a growing field, currently known as "Personalized Medicine." Drugs are being developed that will inhibit certain pathways found in tumor cells.

Many people expect worse side effects from chemotherapy than actually occur. In fact, most side effects can be prevented or greatly reduced.

Nausea and vomiting can nearly always be completely eliminated. Ask the doctor to detail the expected side effects after enumerating the possible side effects. Many patients are able to work and perform most or all of their normal activities while receiving chemotherapy.

GENE THERAPY: Gene therapy has a particular application to cancer because there is a strong genetic basis to many cancers. Cancers grow and spread due, largely, to a mutation in their genes. The cancer cells' mutations may make them invisible to the immune system so they can't be rejected, or the mutations may take away the growth controls built into all cells resulting in uncontrolled growth. Gene therapy examines the genetic content of the cancer cell to see where the defect is, allowing the doctor to choose a drug to target and correct the defect, or cause the cancer cell to die.

Gene therapy is commonly used today. A drug called 'Gleevec' (imatinib) rearranges the two chromosomes, getting rid of the Philadelphia chromosome that causes Chronic Myelogenous Leukemia (CML), putting it into remission. Herceptin (trastuzumab) and Tarceva (erlotinib) target the Epidermal Growth Factor Receptor. The cell cannot stimulate the nucleus to grow and reproduce. Avastin (bevacizumab) targets the Vascular Endothelial Growth Factor Receptor, making it impossible for the cell to stimulate growth of new blood vessels. There are many new drugs in the "pipeline" that target genes or intracellular structures to stop the growth of cancer.

The most highly developed approach to cancer gene therapy is the use of genetically-modified cancer cells as vaccines. The patient's tumor is removed, the cancer cells extracted and grown in a culture. Using the patient's own cells, a vaccine is made. When the patient is vaccinated, the patient makes antibodies toward their cancer cells.

RADIATION THERAPY: As a result of technical advances and training programs, radiation oncology has developed into a highly refined specialty. Now, with superb accuracy, a radiation beam can be focused on the tumor without damaging surrounding normal tissue. By itself, as well as in combination with other therapies, radiation therapy is an increasingly potent tool.

Radiation therapy, in contrast to what many people imagine, does not destroy or dissolve cancer cells like a laser beam would. Its prime mission is to damage the DNA of a malignant cell. The cell does not die instantly, but when it tries to divide, it is unable to and dies at that time. Therefore, radiation treatments continue to have an effect on the tumor after the treatments are completed, often for 90 days and more. Sometimes, tumors shrink primarily after the therapy is finished.

Radiation treatments are normally given five days a week, not because the doctors don't like to work on weekends or have a strong union, but because during the other two days, normal healthy cells will repair some of the damage done to their DNA. Cancerous cells are unable to repair this damage.

Because scar tissue will continue to build up, changes could be noticed in follow-up X-rays even though the tumor is gone. Also, no changes may be noticed in a bone scan for some time, even though the radiation did its job, because the bone mending itself after radiation will give the same image as a tumor on a scan. PET scans can usually distinguish between scar tissue and actively growing tissue.

PROTON THERAPY: As a result of technical advances, *radiation oncology* has developed into a highly refined specialty. Now with superb accuracy, a radiation beam can be focused on the tumor with minimal damage to surrounding normal tissue. It is used to treat cancers in the head and neck and in organs such as the brain, eye, lung, spine, prostate, and deeply seated organs once considered too difficult to treat.

Proton Therapy uses high-energy proton beams which, unlike photon/X-ray beams, are made of protons. Protons are atomic particles found in the nucleus of atoms. With energy generated by a cyclotron, these small particles can be broken loose and aimed directly at the tumor. They are particles with weight and mass, so they have the advantage of depositing most of their energy in the tumor and releasing their energy in a related phenomenon called Bragg Peak. This burst of energy damages the tumor cells' DNA. Proton Therapy reduces the dose to healthy tissues even further. It uses a much different type of beam than photon radiation and permits much deeper penetration while affecting much better control. The necessity of breaking apart the hydrogen atom to form the proton beam requires the energy of a cyclotron, which delivers much more power than the conventional linear accelerators used for CyberKnife, Novalis,

Gamma Knife, etc., can generate. This newly developing technology has limited availability but is becoming more common.

IMMUNIZATION THERAPY: Some of the most exciting possibilities are offered by drugs that work in entirely different ways from the conventional chemotherapy agents. Immunotherapy uses drugs that cause the body's immune system to attack cancer just as it fights off infections. The concept is based on two theories. First, cancer cells can be perceived by the immune system as "foreign" and, with proper help, rejected. The second is that cancer victims have weakened immune systems so that boosting their immune system will help them.

The widely publicized drug, Interferon, stemmed from immunological research. Discovered in the 1950s, it is a protein produced by the body's cells to help fight off viral infections. In cancer, researchers think it fastens onto cells and causes the release of chemicals that inhibit growth. And, because it is a natural substance, experts hoped side effects would be limited. However, we now know that 100% of people taking Interferon will get flu-like symptoms with fever and fatigue. Until the late 1980s, large scale testing of Interferon was not possible because it could be extracted only in minute quantities and at great cost from donated white blood cells. The emergence of recombinant DNA technology, in which common bacteria can be programmed genetically to manufacture quantities of proteins, has made it possible to obtain enough Interferon for cancer research.

On December 5, 1985, the *New England Journal of Medicine* carried a story on Dr. Steve Rosenberg's treatment of Interleukin II combined with LAK cells. That started a torrent of publicity throughout the winter of 1985-1986. Simply stated, this treatment took the natural killer cells from a patient's blood, treated them with IL-2, and reinjected them and more IL-2 back into the patient. These IL-2 armed white cells, called LAK or lymphokine-activated "killer cells," destroy tumors for months after administration in some cases.

Only patients who had failed all other treatments were accepted for this protocol. The success in reducing tumor burden by 50% or more was striking in several types of advanced cancer. In February, 1986, we received a report that Dr. Rosenberg had been successful in 100% (6 out of 6) of the cases of renal cell cancer and 50% (5 out of 10) of the cases of advanced malignant melanoma. Both of these types of cancer were relatively untreatable using other methods of treatment if surgery failed.

The most exciting aspect of this treatment is that IL-2 is not intended to harm the malignant cells. It is solely to stimulate the patient's own immune system which in turn destroys the cancer. Surgery, radiation or chemotherapy, the methods of treatment most physicians are used to discussing in fighting cancer, are each designed to damage malignant cells in their own way. The mere concept of IL-2, as well as the success of the treatments, emphasizes the importance of the patient's immune system. Since 1986, this form of therapy has been used in fighting cancer.

It seems that there are a number of substances that occur naturally in the body to maintain normal growth and development which may be utilized to stimulate the body's natural defenses against cancer. The National Cancer Institute has established a special research program to explore intensively the therapeutic applications of these naturally occurring substances called "Biological Response Modifiers."

HYPERTHERMIA: This is the process of heating a tumor from 98.6° up to 113° Fahrenheit.

Hyperthermia is given with chemotherapy or radiation therapy because it is not effective by itself. It can magnify the benefits of chemotherapy or radiation therapy several fold without much downside risk. This in and of itself is capable of killing certain types of cancer. Heated Intraperitoneal Chemotherapy is different. After the tumor is removed as much as possible, chemotherapy, warmed to 109.4°, is pumped into the open abdomen and bathes the tissues for a period of time. When the chemotherapy solution is drained from the site, the patient's surgical incision is closed. This technique positively affects survival in patients with difficult-to-treat abdominal tumors.

Radio Frequency Ablation is another form of hyperthermia done by inserting a special needle into a tumor. The physician is guided in the placement of the needle by images from an imaging machine, such as a CT scanner. Once the needle is in place, tines are deployed from the hollow core of the needle. These tines penetrate and envelope the tumor. RFA energy is then sent through the needle and tines, destroying the tumor. This technique can be used for tumors of the liver, bone, kidney, and lung. Whether or not this technique is used depends on the location and size of the tumor.

HORMONAL MANIPULATION: The art of treating certain cancers by denying needed hormones, hormonal manipulation is normally one of the more pleasant treatments as it is non-toxic and has very minimal side effects. Its use is tested regularly for treatment of breast cancer. If applicable, it is certainly a treatment of choice and can be used along with other forms of therapy.

A pathologist described it in a fascinating way. A malignant cell is examined and found to be estrogen or progesterone positive, meaning it is dependent on those substances for survival. There is a door on the side of each malignant cell that opens to allow those substances to enter. By giving a certain pill, those doors are sealed shut and the malignant cells are deprived of this hormone they need to survive and divide and are killed. Sometimes, surgery is needed to remove the gland that makes a certain hormone. Hormonal manipulation is also called endocrine therapy, hormonal therapy, and hormone treatment.

PHOTODYNAMIC THERAPY: Photo-dynamic Therapy was developed at Roswell Park Memorial Institute in Buffalo, New York in the early 1970s. It has been on the periphery of cancer treatment since that time, and used for tumors of the esophagus and non-small-cell lung cancer. A patient getting this type of treatment is first injected with a photosensitizing drug, HPPH. Twenty-four to sixty hours later, the drug has circulated enough to have concentrated itself in the tumor, but not in healthy cells. The patient is taken to the treatment room and a scope with a laser is passed to the level of the tumor. The laser is pulsed and the tumor dies as a result of the exposure to light. Because healthy cells can excrete the photosensitizer more easily than the cancer cells, there are few side effects. The biggest drawback to this therapy is that the light does not penetrate more than ten millimeters, so tumors have to be small in order to have any benefit. Since many tumors of the esophagus and lung are diagnosed at a later stage, this treatment is very seldom used. Clinical trials are examining potential use for brain, skin, prostate, cervix, liver, and abdominal cavity cancers.

MONOCLONAL ANTIBODIES: Monoclonal antibodies target a single receptor on a cell. These drugs, when they bind to the cell, program the cell to die or mark it for destruction by other cells. The surfaces of viruses, bacteria and even normal cells contain specific molecules that are called antigens. When they enter the body, these antigens or T-cells (fighter cells) trigger the B-cells (also fighter cells) which then turn into an antibody-producing factory. Antibodies attach to the invading cells, causing their destruction. All vaccines are made from antigens that induce the formation of antibodies in advance to ward off infectious diseases. These drugs include rituximab, trastuzumab, and bevacizumab.

To develop antibodies, mice are injected with antigens, for example, human cancer cells. The mouse then makes antibodies to different components of the cancer cells, including abnormal proteins associated with cancer itself. The mouse's spleen, where much of the antibody production occurs, is removed and its cells extracted. These cells are then fused with cancer cells from another mouse with myeloma. These tumor cells are used because they are immortal: they will continue to divide ad infinitum and make the fused hybrid do the same. Finally, the hybrid cells that are producing the particular antibodies they want, are selected and encouraged to reproduce, or clone, in separate tissue cultures. All of this is done in the laboratory. The products are called monoclonal antibodies because each comes from a single line, or clone, of cells.

Special antigens can be found on some cancer cells that are not present on normal cells. Lab-produced antibodies home in on tumors like heat-seeking missiles while ignoring normal tissue. These antibodies are tagged with radioactive substances or chemicals to carry lethal doses directly to cancer cells while bypassing normal cells. When the antibodies connect to cells, the radioisotope is unlocked, causing a bigger cell death.

COMMON CANCER TERMS
IN LAY LANGUAGE

Adjuvant treatment. Treatments to fight cancer when there is no physical evidence of remaining cancer in the body.

Benign. Cells forming a tumor that are not presently cancerous and cannot spread from their original site and reach the blood stream or lymphatic system.

Biopsy. The examination of tissue to determine whether it is malignant or benign.

Cancer. The uncontrolled growth of malignant cells.

Carcinogen. A cancer-causing substance.

Carcinoma. A malignant tumor arising in the sheets of cells covering the surface of the body and lining of various glands.

Chemotherapy. Treatment through the use of chemicals.

Immunization Therapy. Treatment by activating the immune system.

Leukemia. Cancer arising in the blood-forming cells of the bone marrow.

Lymphoma. Cancer arising in the lymph nodes.

Malignant. Cells which will continue to grow geometrically and are considered cancerous.

Metastasize. The breaking away of cancer cells from the original tumor, settling elsewhere in the body and forming a new tumor.

Nuclear Medicine. Another term for scans or tomagrams.

Oncologist. A doctor specializing in the treatment of cancer. He may further specialize in medicine, radiation or surgery, but always in relation to cancer.

Palliative Treatment. Treatment that relieves pain and symptoms but is not intended to cure disease.

Pathology. The examination of tissues and body fluids to determine whether malignant cells are present and to ascertain the type or origin of these cells.

Prognosis. The projected future course of the illness.

Protocol. A specific treatment or series of treatments that has been developed to treat cancer.

Radiotherapy. Treatment by the use of radiation or X-rays.

Recurrence. The return of cancer after it was thought to be in remission or cured.

Remission. When cancer can no longer be found to be present but cannot be determined as cured.

Sarcoma. A malignant tumor arising in supporting structures such as fibrous tissue and blood vessels.

Scan. A picture of a particular part of the body, such as bones, brain or liver, produced by counting the radiation caused by radioactive particles being absorbed by that part of the body.

Tomogram. A computer-produced vertical X-ray capable of giving continuous "vertical slices" of various parts of the body.

Tumor. The mass caused by a concentration of cells, either benign or malignant.

ONE DAY AT A TIME

There are two days in every week about which you should not worry; two days which should be kept free from fear and apprehension.

One of these is YESTERDAY with its mistakes and cares, its faults and blunders, its aches and pains. Yesterday has passed forever beyond our control. All the money in the world cannot bring back yesterday. We cannot undo a single act we performed; we cannot erase a single word said. Yesterday is gone!

The other day we should not worry about is TOMORROW, with its possible burden, its large promise and poor performance. Tomorrow is also beyond our immediate control. Tomorrow's sun will rise, either in splendor or behind a mask of clouds - but it will rise. Until it does, we have no stake in tomorrow, for it is yet unborn.

This leaves only one day - TODAY! Any man can fight the battle of just one day. It is only when you and I have the burdens in these two awful extremities - yesterday and tomorrow - that we break down.

It is not the experience of today that drives men mad. It is the remorse or bitterness about something which happened yesterday and the dread of what tomorrow may bring.

LET US THEREFORE LIVE
BUT ONLY ONE DAY AT A TIME.

~ Author unknown ~

14 Plaques on the Positive Mental Attitude Walk at the Richard and Annette Bloch Cancer Survivors Parks

1. Cancer is the most curable of all chronic diseases.

2. There are treatments for every type of cancer.

3. Some people have been cured from every type of cancer.

4. There are 11,000,000 living Americans who have been diagnosed with cancer; 6,000,000 are considered cured.

5. Realize that cancer is a life threatening disease but some beat it. Make up your mind you will be one of those who do.

6. Make a commitment to do everything in your power to help yourself fight the disease.

7. Find a qualified doctor in whom you have confidence who believes he can successfully treat you.

8. Regardless of the prognosis, get an independent qualified second opinion.

9. Treat your cancer promptly, properly and thoroughly and have a positive mental attitude.

10. Get PDQ from 1-800-4-CANCER.
    Know all your options. Knowledge heals.

11. Seek and accept support.

12. Have plans for pleasant things to do and
    goals to accomplish.

13. Read and practice suggestions in
    Fighting Cancer available free from
    1-800-433-0464.

14. Make up your mind that when your
    cancer is gone, you are through with it.

Road to Recovery Plaques

CANCER

Cancer is the uncontrolled growth of cells. Even though it is not the largest killer, it is the most feared disease in America because it is not understood. If we understood cancer, we would not be as afraid of it. It is estimated that the average individual has a wildly dividing cell six times a day. The immune system recognizes this, kills it, and we never know the difference. When the immune system lets down, even temporarily, and these dividing cells get established to the point that the immune system cannot control them, we have cancer.

COMMITMENT

The biggest and the hardest single thing that you will be required to do in the entire battle is to make up your mind to really fight it. You must, on your own, make the commitment that you will do everything in your power to fight your disease. No exceptions. Nothing halfway. Nothing for the sake of ease or convenience. Everything! Nothing short of it. When you have done this, you have accomplished the most difficult thing you will have to accomplish throughout your entire treatment.

KNOWLEDGE

Knowledge is a cancer patient's best friend. The more you know about your disease, the better your chances are of beating it. Find out everything you can about your disease. Knowledge heals; ignorance kills. Read the book *Fighting Cancer*, available free from 800-433-0464 or www.blochcancer.org.

TREATMENTS

Find a qualified physician who believes you can be successfully treated. Get an independent second opinion to be certain you are doing everything possible correctly. Do everything your physician suggests and do everything you believe might help that your physician says will not hurt. You are the boss. This is your life.

PHYSICAL WELFARE

Eat a well-balanced diet to maintain an effective immune system. Do not go on any fad diets at this time. Exercise as much as you comfortably can. Be selfish, think of yourself first, and do not overdo.

MENTAL WELFARE

There are many mental exercises that could help your recovery and cannot possibly hurt.

Relaxation exercises are strongly recommended as stress accelerates cancer growth. Visual imagery has been demonstrated to improve the chances of success. Prayer by individuals unknown to the patient have been clinically demonstrated to improve the chances of success, so prayers by the patient could certainly help and cannot hurt. Make certain your attitude is receptive to successful treatment and keep a positive outlook.

SUMMARY

Fighting cancer is not a simple matter of thinking positively, wishing it away and saying, "Hey, doc, cure me." It is a matter of educating yourself about every detail and mustering all your resources. Use every drop of energy in an organized fashion to constructively concentrate on getting rid of cancer.

Most cancers can be successfully treated, but generally you have only one chance. If you miss that first chance, if you don't do everything in your power, often there is no second chance. This is why no cancer patient can afford the luxury of looking back and saying, "I wish I would have...." Never look back. Concentrate on this moment forward and do everything in your power. There is no downside risk. Now you may have a chance.

Part III   For Casual Supporters

This chapter is written specifically for the friend, neighbor, business associate or anyone wishing to have contact with the patient other than the primary supporter.

Nearly everyone is touched by someone they know getting cancer. The universal reaction is one of helplessness. "I don't know what to say." "I don't know what to do." The following will help you be constructive and show your concern.

Let the patient know you are thinking about them. Do not procrastinate. Life is not a dress rehearsal. This is the main performance. It is now, as soon as you hear about the problem, that the patient needs to know of your concern and caring. Visit the patient even if you feel uncomfortable.

Regardless of the prognosis, the patient is still a human being with the same likes and dislikes as before the diagnosis. Their focus may have changed, but their interests remain the same. They should not be treated as a leper – they are not contagious. They should not be neglected or ignored.

The most comfortable way to approach them is to be natural, be open, talk about their problem and be as normal in your conversation as always. Avoiding the subject and being hush-hush causes more stress and strain with everyone involved. Use the word cancer - call it what it is.

Be totally honest with any discussions. Never lie or state anything that is not a fact. For example, never say, "I know you are going to get well." You can't possibly know that. On the other hand, do not think of the patient as being hopeless. Your feelings have a way of coming through. Any conversation with the patient about the future of their disease should be expressed as optimistically as possible. For example, "I read about great progress being made with new discoveries and new treatments." "You have so many things going for you," etc. is so much more optimistic than saying, "So many people die from this disease."

Never compare the patient with anyone else. Don't give advice on new treatments and certainly don't recommend alternative therapies such as laetrile, macrobiotic diets, etc. No two cases of cancer are the same. No two people are the same. Treatments, side effects or results for one patient can be completely different for another.

Talk about past occasions and achievements and reminisce about good times. Let them know how they have been special and meaningful in your life. Don't be afraid to be funny and laugh. Laughter is therapeutic. Don't be afraid to cry with the patient and family. It can lead to meaningful conversations.

Possibly the most important word is listen. The burden of conversation will not be entirely on your shoulders. Hear and comprehend what the patient is truly saying. Share your feelings and thoughts about their concerns.

The following is a list of suggestions:

→ Visit the patient promptly.

→ Do grocery shopping.

→ Ask what you can do to help.

→ Offer to stay with the patient, so the caretaker can get out.

→ Give books of short stories. Paperback books are easier to hold.

→ Offer special invitations even if they can't come. They will feel included and less isolated. Include the patient and family in your activities.

→ Do not visit if you have a cold or the flu. Their immune system might be weakened from treatments.

→ Don't be afraid to use the word cancer – call it what it is.

➡ Make it clear that you are with the patient to help and give support, not to offer sympathy. Be calm and just be there.

➡ Be a good listener.

➡ If the patient expresses feelings of being a burden, reassure them by saying you have chosen freely to be there.

➡ Treat the patient as if you expect them to live. You need not believe they *will*, you only need believe they *can* recover.

➡ Have patience. Not everyone hears the information the first time.

➡ Don't be afraid to cry with the patient and family. This can lead to meaningful conversations.

➡ Don't tell them to keep a stiff upper lip or keep smiling. You can say it must be very hard or very tiring or very frightening.

➡ Allow them to express anger when it is to relieve stress.

➡ Express love, caring and concern verbally and through actions at every opportunity. Letters, cards and flowers are tangible methods.

→ Cancer is not contagious. Touch, hug, kiss. Human contact is very necessary.

→ The patient needs reassurance that you care for them even though their physical appearance might have changed.

→ Give them something special they might not want to buy for themself.

→ Provide companionship with the patient during meals and other appropriate times.

→ Be cheerful whenever you are around the patient. Being depressed and gloomy is contagious, and the patient could catch it.

→ Be completely honest with the patient.

→ Keep no secrets from the patient.

→ Do not whisper to others in front of the patient.

→ Think of the patient as an individual, a unique human being, not a statistic.

→ Discuss all the normal things with the patient that they have always been interested in. While cancer might have become the dominant item in their life, their interests have not changed.

→ Encourage the patient to believe that their actions could make a difference in the outcome and the quality of their life.

→ Make no prognosis. It can only cast doubts on your credibility.

→ Encourage the patient to learn everything about their cancer that they can.

→ If the patient has adverse side effects from treatments, encourage them to realize what it is doing to those weak cancer cells.

→ True love is never having to say "I'm sorry." Erase that phrase from your vocabulary. Sympathize with them, not for them.

→ Advise the patient that you are saying prayers for them and urge them to say prayers for themselves.

→ Do not assume the patient is going to die. Many are cured.

→ Record messages, favorite music or books.

→ Share your feelings with the children. Help them talk and share their feelings.

→ Encourage them to keep as physically and mentally active as they are capable.

→ Don't be afraid to be funny and laugh. Laughter is therapy. Watch funny movies. Give joke books.

→ Do not tell horror stories of other cancer patients.

→ Talk about past occasions and reminisce about good times. Discuss how they have been special and meaningful to your life.

→ Never discourage an optimistic outlook.

→ Provide pedicure, manicure, hair stylist or pretty scarves – anything to build their self-esteem.

→ Give a make-up lesson or gentle massage.

→ Do not encourage the patient to try alternative therapies.

You are a concerned and caring person, as evidenced by the fact that you are reading this book. Let the patient know you are thinking about them as soon as you learn about their problem. The longer you put it off, the more difficult it will be. The diagnosis of cancer is so devastating, the patient needs all the love and support you can give to see them through the difficult days. Just remember to be natural and let your relationship be as it was. They are the same individual as they were before the diagnosis. Let them know you are available. You will both be better for it.

About the Authors

Richard A. (Dick) Bloch, born in Kansas City, Missouri on February 15, 1926, was the youngest of three sons. An entrepreneur at heart, at age nine he bought a hand printing press and started a business. He was so successful that by his twelfth birthday, he had progressed to three automatic presses and was doing much of the printing for all the high schools in Kansas City. After high school, he sold his business to a college in Iowa as a model shop for use in printing courses.

Dick attended the Wharton School of Finance at the University of Pennsylvania where he received a bachelor of science degree in economics at the age of 19. While in college, he bought cars, took them apart, put them back together and then sold them to pay for his expenses. After graduation, Bloch joined his older brother, Henry, in the formation of a bookkeeping and tax preparation company. They started a new company in 1955 specializing in just tax preparation, H&R Block, Inc. Today H&R Block operates more than 11,000 offices worldwide and prepares over 24,000,000 income tax returns annually.

In 1978, Dick was told he had terminal lung cancer with three months to live. Refusing to accept this prognosis, he went to a major comprehensive cancer center where, after two years of aggressive therapy, he was told he was cured. After Dick's bout with cancer, he focused his attention on working "to help the next person who gets cancer." He sold his interest in H&R Block, Inc. and retired from the company in 1982 to be able to devote all his efforts to cancer. To do this, he and Annette, his wife, formed the R.A. Bloch Cancer Foundation.

Richard and Annette Bloch are founders of the Cancer Hot Line in Kansas City, a volunteer organization that matches cancer patients with a survivor of that type of cancer. The Cancer Hotline has received more than 200,000 calls from newly diagnosed cancer patients since its inception in 1980.

They also founded the R.A. Bloch Cancer Management Center at the University of Missouri-Kansas City. This was a free multi-disciplinary second opinion panel staffed from 1980 to 1995 by over 100 physicians donating their time to help some 250 cancer patients per year know they were receiving the best possible treatment. Because of greatly increased demand, it was closed and replaced by local institutions offering a similar service.

On May 1, 1988, the R. A. Bloch Cancer Support Center was dedicated on the grounds of the University of Missouri – Kansas City. It was a relaxing, comfortable place for patients and their supporters to congregate for the purposes of sharing and education. This was coordinated by professionals and like all other Bloch programs, completely free. Innovative support programs were developed at the Center and sent out into the community. Once these programs were established throughout the area, they felt that it was no longer necessary to maintain the facility. The Support Center closed in 2001.

Dick conceived of a computer program which the National Cancer Institute implemented under the name "PDQ" for "Physicians Data Query." It gives the state-of-the-art treatment for every type and stage of cancer and all the current clinical trials. This information is gathered from every cancer center in the United States and over 22 foreign countries and is continuously updated by a staff of 108 researchers. In government publications it states, "If physicians avail themselves of the opportunity now offered by PDQ, the NCI estimates the national survival rates would rise by at least 10% or more than

40,000 lives per year." The government named the building housing this program in Bethesda, MD the R.A. Bloch International Cancer Information Center.

Dick and Annette are the authors of three books. CANCER...*there's hope* is a story of Richard and Annette's fight against his "terminal" lung cancer. It is written, not to tell a story, but to show others what they can do to battle this disease. *Fighting Cancer* is a step-by-step guide for cancer patients to help themselves fight the disease. *Guide for Cancer Supporters* is written to help supporters exclusively. All three are available free by calling the Bloch Cancer Hot Line at 800-433-0464 or from our website at www.blochcancer.org.

Dick and Annette started the Fighting Cancer Rally in 1986 to demonstrate that death and cancer are not synonymous, and there is a possibility of a quality of life after the diagnosis of cancer. Over 700 Cancer Survivor Day Rallies now are held across the United States and in over 15 countries on the first Sunday in June.

At the Rally in Kansas City in June 1990, the first R.A. Bloch Cancer Survivors Park was dedicated to the 5,000,000 living Americans who had been diagnosed with cancer, 2,000,000 of whom were considered cured. Today those figures have more than doubled!

In addition to Kansas City, other Richard and Annette Bloch Cancer Survivors Parks have been completed in Bakersfield, CA; Baltimore, MD; Chicago, IL; Cleveland, OH; Columbia, SC; Columbus, OH; Dallas, TX; Houston, TX; Indianapolis, IN; Jacksonville, FL; Memphis, TN; Minneapolis, MN; Mississauga, Ontario, Canada; New Orleans, LA; Omaha, NE; Ottawa, Ontario, Canada; Phoenix, AZ; Rancho Mirage, CA; Sacramento, CA; San Diego, CA, Santa Rosa, CA; Tucson, AZ, and Tampa, FL.

Annette and Dick talked to over 1,000 cancer patients individually each year, listening to their problems and trying to help them and their families. They went around the country speaking to different groups and organizations. They have been the subject of articles in numerous magazines including Family Circle, Medical World News, People, Cosmopolitan, Vogue, and Reader's Digest. They have appeared on national television on every major network and in numerous documentaries. They have received awards or been honored by such organizations as the American Cancer Society, the Sertoma Club, the Department of Health and Human Services, the Rotary Club, the Lion's Club, Church of Jesus Christ of Latter-day Saints, and they received the Mankind Award from Cystic Fibrosis.

In 1982, Dick was appointed by President Reagan to the National Cancer Advisory Board for a 6-year term. In 1989, he was selected as one of the "Most Caring Individuals" from 4,000 nominees by the Caring Institute in Washington. He was a member of the President's Circle of the National Academy of Sciences, the Institute of Medicine and was on the NIH's Office of Alternative Medicine for two years. Dick received the American Society of Clinical Oncology's Public Service Award in 1994 in recognition of exemplary contributions to the field of oncology and to patients with cancer. He received the 1995 Layman's Award from the Society of Surgical Oncology at their Annual Convention. Also in 1995, Dick and Annette received Coping Magazine's 1995 Hero Award for Lifetime Achievement. In 2003, Dick was honored as the first recipient of the Allesandro di Montezemolo Lifetime Achievement Award given by the American-Italian Cancer Foundation for his dedication to helping cancer patients, especially the development of PDQ. Dick died in 2004 of heart failure.

Annette Modell Bloch was born in Philadelphia, Pennsylvania where she lived until her marriage to Richard Bloch. She and Dick have three daughters, seven grandchildren, and seven great grandchildren. A breast cancer survivor and philanthropist, Annette is president of the R.A. Bloch Cancer Foundation and oversees the Bloch Cancer Hotline. She is a trustee of the Palm Springs Art Museum. She received the Palm Springs, California Chamber of Commerce's Athena Award for her commitment to helping others. Also in Palm Springs, she has received a Meritorious Gold Palm Star for her enduring and selfless contributions to charitable causes. Annette's work on behalf of heart and cancer patients has established the Richard and Annette Bloch Heart Rhythm Center, the Richard and Annette Bloch Cancer Care Pavilion and the Richard and Annette Bloch Radiation Oncology Pavilion at the University of Kansas Hospital in Kansas City as well as the Annette Bloch Cancer Care Center for the Desert AIDS Project in Palm Springs, California.

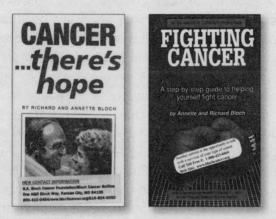

CANCER...*there's hope*
Explaining in lay terms what cancer is and
what a patient can do to help themself.

FIGHTING CANCER
A step-by-step guide to help patients to help
themselves fight cancer.

**Printed and audio versions
are available free
by calling
1-800-433-0464
or on the web at
www.blochcancer.org**

NOTES: